EBURY PRESS
THE DRY FASTING MIRACLE

Luke Coutinho is a globally renowned holistic lifestyle coach and an award-winning holistic nutritionist. He is the co-author of the bestsellers *The Great Indian Diet* and *The Magic Weight-Loss Pill*.

Sheikh Abdulaziz Bin Ali Bin Rashed Al Nuaimi, better known as the 'Green Sheikh', is a member of the Ajman royal family in the United Arab Emirates. His Highness has made a name for himself as one of the most resilient and vocal proponents of the environment.

PRAISE FOR THE BOOK

'Hey Luke, I was bulimic, with no control over emotional eating. I had severe arthritis pain . . . All that vanished, thanks to your advice. Dry fasting is ultimate. I am planning to ask my teenage girls to follow dry fasting as well . . . Thank you and god bless you. It feels great to be in control'—Sherina Nair

'Hi Luke! I don't know if this happened because of dry fasting, but I believe it did. I am a home baker and December was a crazy month for me. So much so that on 1 January my body crashed. I had acute pain in the back and the legs. No amount of painkillers helped. I got a lady masseuse and that helped a bit. However, I started dry fasting this week, for about fifteen hours a day and with two meals a day, and started going for a walk. My masseuse came again today and couldn't believe my recovery. A girl who was howling in pain at the slightest touch and pressure was just fine. I still have a little pain in one spot but I am otherwise perfect. The knots in my legs have almost vanished. Not only that, in four days, she says my legs have visibly slimmed. Thank you so much for all that you are doing so selflessly to make us a healthy lot. Stay blessed, and may you soar higher and higher!'—Saryu Bansal

'Ever since I have had the pleasure of being part of your team, I have tried to follow the practise-what-you-preach policy. It's been five months now, and I see myself as a changed person. I was someone who would faint without tea and breakfast, but over the past three months, I have completely given up drinking my morning tea. And not one day have I got a headache! Because I had told myself that I would be fine. I started with intermittent fasting and, slowly, as I got the hang of it, breakfast didn't seem to be the most important meal of my day! Not once did I feel dizzy. And today I dry-fasted for sixteen hours. I feel light, I feel amazing—like I have won a battle. From being someone who could never miss breakfast to this—I'm so happy (and maybe just a little bit proud) that I'm no longer dependent on anything. I have lost a few inches too. Post delivery, it wasn't easy losing weight. My husband was pleasantly surprised. I'm trying to rediscover the girl in myself. Thank you so much, from the bottom of my heart. May god bless you'—Dr Manali

'The first magical effect of dry fasting has been on my chronic pain. Dear readers, just wanted to share with you all that I have been suffering from cervical muscular pain for the past seven years. A lot of medication and physiotherapy has been done. My daily routine had been dependent on Omnigel or Moov. I used to have to take painkillers at least twice a week. My belief was that if I missed any meal, I would get a headache—and it's true in my case. I was fed up with my lifestyle and wanted change. So now I have been dry-fasting for thirteen–seventeen hours a day for the past twenty days, for three–four days a week. Today I didn't have to apply Omnigel, and it feels great. I feel more active. I also feel a lot less pain. I can easily survive by skipping meals and water. It's no less than a miracle for me. I have observed some weight loss too. It's a win-win situation for me. I am so glad. All thanks go to this group and our mentor, Luke Coutinho. With a lot of gratitude and regards'—Purnima Goley Singh

'Hi Luke—gratitude. I have been practising dry fasting for months now on a regular basis. A few months back, I felt an unknown pain in my hip bones. I got X-rays done, but there seemed to be nothing serious about it—just low levels of vitamins D and B12. But even after being on medication, the pain didn't go away. After I started dry fasting, my condition is far, far better, and last week I went gluten- and dairy-free for three days, and now it's completely gone. I feel more relaxed now . . . I have made one more lifestyle change, along with adding dry fasting to my routine—I will go gluten- and dairy-free twice a week. Thank you for showing us the better part of us hidden within'—Anjali Garg

'Hi Luke, I realized recently that the most uncomfortable phase in a woman's life is early menopause. I get irritated easily, and the hormones saddled me with depression and mood swings. It was at this point that you spoke to me about a three-day global dry fasting period. I have only gratitude for you today—thank you very much. Since then, I have been dry-fasting for two days a week and have been practising intermittent fasting for the rest of the days. I am yet to strictly follow many things that this routine needs me to, but today I am so happy that on my twenty-second marriage anniversary, I could comfortably fit into my seven-year-old top, which has always been one of my favourites. People just say that we should stay healthy, but you ensure that we don't lose inspiration, as your daily videos work like medicine for us. And I would like to say to my Sangha community— each one of you have inspired me'—Padma Nalini

ALSO BY LUKE COUTINHO

The Great Indian Diet
The Magic Weight-Loss Pill

THE DRY FASTING MIRACLE

FROM DEPRIVE TO THRIVE

LUKE COUTINHO AND
SHEIKH ABDULAZIZ BIN ALI BIN RASHED AL NUAIMI

EBURY
PRESS

An imprint of Penguin Random House

EBURY PRESS

USA | Canada | UK | Ireland | Australia
New Zealand | India | South Africa | China

Ebury Press is part of the Penguin Random House group of companies
whose addresses can be found at global.penguinrandomhouse.com

Published by Penguin Random House India Pvt. Ltd
7th Floor, Infinity Tower C, DLF Cyber City,
Gurgaon 122 002, Haryana, India

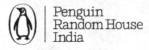

Penguin
Random House
India

First published in Ebury Press by Penguin Random House India 2020

10 9 8 7 6 5 4 3 2 1

The views and opinions expressed in this book are the authors' own and the facts
are as reported by them, which have been verified to the extent possible, and the
publishers are not in any way liable for the same. Neither the authors nor the
publishers of *The Dry Fasting Miracle* are doctors or medical care providers and
have no expertise in diagnosing, examining or treating medical conditions of any
kind, or in determining the effect of any specific exercise on a medical condition. The
information and exercises provided in this book are for reference only and are to be
used under professional guidance. They are not offered as a replacement or substitute
for professional medical advice or treatment. Not all diets are suitable for everyone,
and making use of this or any other diet injudiciously may result in injury.

Always, in your particular case, consult a doctor and obtain full medical clearance
before practising any diet. The authors, publishers and distributors assume no
responsibility or liability for any injuries or losses that may result from practising
any diet, or from the adoption of any instruction or advice expressed in this book.
The authors, publishers and distributors make no representations or warranties with
regards to the completeness or accuracy of information contained in this book.

No part of this book is meant or intended to be a substitute for medicine or any
treatment you are undergoing. Always seek advice from your doctor before starting
any fast.

ISBN 9780143450894

Typeset in Sabon by Manipal Technologies Limited, Manipal

www.penguin.co.in

I dedicate this book to all of humanity
Luke Coutinho

I dedicate this book to Allah the Almighty
Sheikh Abdulaziz Bin Ali Bin Rashed Al Nuaimi

CONTENTS

FOREWORD

By Taarika Dave

Thank you, Luke, for giving me the opportunity to contribute to this book. *The Dry Fasting Miracle* is a boon for so many people who know about fasting but have a lot of confusion around the many fads associated with it. The book helps answer all queries, and clarify concepts and wrong beliefs around dry fasting in the simplest manner possible. With so much positive feedback around dry fasting, it gives me immense pleasure to be writing about this one lifestyle change that has transformed the lives of so many people across the world.

While fasting has been part of our lifestyle from even before you and I existed, over the years we have forgotten about it. There are a couple of reasons that can be attributed to this:

- 24x7 availability of food.
- The faulty concept that eating small quantities and frequently will lead to high metabolism.
- Boredom and emotional eating.

- Fad diets, which fail at giving what our body needs at a cellular level for health and immunity.

Every day Luke and his team, which includes me, wake up to so many inspiring stories of people—including our clients—sharing their experiences of fasting. While some have gotten rid of arthritic pain, some have experienced a boost in their immunity and haven't fallen sick over a long period of time; some have had their headaches and migraines go away while some have noticed a drastic improvement in their quality of sleep and energy levels. And there are those who have just fallen in love with the way their skin and hair have improved because of fasting.

Fasting is the way to good health from here on. It's no longer about what we can add to boost our health—it's about what can we reduce or eliminate. We are eating way more than our bodies are designed to handle. Not to forget our mostly sedentary lifestyles. This trend of constantly munching on something has to go. If we could ask our ancestors how much they ate, they would probably tell us how they ate to live, and not lived to eat. We have to honour the body and its needs. While our goals and ambitions in life may have changed with the passing years, our body's basic requirements haven't.

This book isn't aiming at teaching you a new concept. It's aimed at helping you get on a lifestyle path that serves you best. It lays out the basic guidelines of living, for fasting is a way of living and everything is connected to it—right from your digestion, quality of sleep, energy levels, mood, thoughts and detoxification to brain health, bone health, immunity and mental resilience. It is that powerful.

While it has almost been a year of fasting on and off, depending on when my body feels the need to take a break, fasting came most naturally to me when I adopted the circadian-rhythm fasting. You will read more about it in the coming chapters. It has just been fifteen days that I have adopted this, and it changed the way I felt and looked the very next day. Zero bloating, a flat stomach, high energy levels and a feeling of waking up squeaky-clean! I did not adopt fasting to manage any health condition, because, thankfully, I have none; I took it up only for discipline—and that's the crux when it comes to good health. I also did it because I was extremely motivated after hearing some life-changing testimonials from people all over the world. The most magical one was from a lady experiencing her old skin peel off with fasting while new skin made its way in! It was unbelievable for me to hear that. The more I come across such fasting stories, the more I sit back and wonder at the incredible potential our body has when it gets it basics right.

A few takeaways from my own experience:

- Keep fasting simple. It does not have to be complicated. If it is, you are doing it wrong.
- Know that fasting DOES NOT mean starving.
- While the concept of fasting works for most of us, the frequency and duration of it is highly personalized. No one, not even Luke, can tell you how much you

should fast. Your body is going to be your best indicator.

- Please, please, please do not compete with others when it comes to fasting. You will defeat the whole purpose of it.
- Fasting means complete rest to the digestive system. You could, at most, be drinking plain water. Nothing else.
- While keeping fasting challenges is a great idea, do not force anyone into it. Every individual should have the right and the ability to decide when and how to fast.

I promise that if you get all your fasting concepts in place, do it with the right intention and are in tune with your body, fasting can change your life and health completely.

PREFACE

By Luke Coutinho

I would, first, like to thank all my readers for the immense love and support they gave me after the publication of the first version of *The Dry Fasting Miracle*. While selling thousands of copies worldwide, we knew that it would impact the lives of so many people across the world.

When I first sat down to write this book, my only intention was to revive the age-old practice and wisdom of dry fasting and encourage every home to take this up as a lifestyle change. Today, when I look back at the number of testimonials and stories that continue to pour in from people about how dry fasting has been the No. 1 game changer for their health, I feel there is so much that our body is capable of achieving, provided we give it the right set of conditions. While dry fasting is just one practice, its impact and effects are varied. It's amazing how different bodies will respond to this one simple practice in different ways, and the more I see and hear from all of you, the more I learn about the human body.

With the release of the first version of the book, more and more powerful testimonials came in, and this was the motivation behind a newer and better version of *The Dry Fasting Miracle*. The new, revised and updated version is backed by more research and evidence, and we are hoping that the book changes the health of every person who reads it.

Fasting is not something that I have recently discovered, and it certainly isn't a new concept. It is practised in almost every region and religion of the world. Ever since human life existed on this planet, we have, in a way, been fasting, because food was limited and periods of feasting (hunting, in those days) were followed by periods of fasting. Human beings during evolution did not wake up to a shelf full of breakfast cereals and beverages, as we do today. They had to wait for it to get bright and sunny outside so they could set out on the day's hunt and then finally feast, followed by a period of fasting again.

Now consider our lives today. We have entered a global culture of constantly eating, nibbling and snacking, with very little or no fasting involved, unless someone gets sick and the body is forced to fast to heal. Before our body is even done digesting and eliminating the last meal, we are putting more food into our system. When we eat too much, our digestive system has to go on overdrive, which means constantly utilizing the body's energy, producing acids and enzymes. In most cases, we don't even let the process of digestion be completed. Today, there is an abundance of food everywhere; there is overeating and gluttony. Our body was never designed to eat so much food as we do today. We have moved far away from nature and its two cycles—elimination and building.

In the elimination phase, our body is designed to detoxify, clean, repair, rejuvenate and balance out our hormones. In the building phase, we eat to build, create, heal and grow.

But since we are eating throughout the day, our elimination phase has become shorter and building phase longer. Thus, we experience toxic overload, stubborn fat, constant fatigue, hair fall, chronic acidity, etc. Most diseases are caused only by overeating.

In a line, overeating is: More acid secretion; more inflammation; more mucous secretion; the right environment for pathogens to breed.

So how do we deal with the issue? What is the solution? The answer is fasting.

Fasting triggers the body's internal healing mechanism. It's no magic, but the intelligence of our body. You get a cut on your finger and your body's intelligence springs into action to heal the cut by forming a scab. Similarly, you fast and your body's intelligence springs into action to start the healing process. So give your body the foundation it needs to heal, and allow it to do its job.

When we sat down to research dry fasting, we came across numerous studies done on it—for Ramadan in Muslims and Lent in Christians—showing us the importance these religions placed on fasting. One can think that fasting is a spiritual practice. Yes, it is, but it is also so much more.

I advocate dry fasting and intermittent fasting for the body's natural healing and regeneration, and always will, because not only have I experienced its benefits myself, I have also seen my patients, clients and people all over the world experiencing its miracles. Some of them have experienced breakthrough healing, which only makes me wonder anew at our body's immense potential and intelligence.

One of the first questions I come across is: Will fasting suit me?

Well, do it and see. There are as many different outcomes of fasting as the many people who do it. We have to have an open mind to experience its results. Nothing works if you are scared. Fear is the most limiting human emotion. You never know how your body will respond to the gift of fasting. But one thing I can say for sure out of my experience—if fasting is something that suits your body, its outcome will be nothing short of a miracle. Do it the right way, know its concepts and respect your body. That is key.

Dry fasting and intermittent fasting will be the future of preventative healthcare if done the right, smart and intelligent way. It costs no money and is something natural to living beings, including humans. It doesn't have to suit everyone, but if it does suit you, it's a free way of living that can enhance your overall well-being and immunity, improve the quality of your skin and hair, boost your metabolism and energy levels, and increase longevity. It's the inexpensive way to great health.

Get back to nature, my friends. Get back to a diet and eating pattern that was designed by nature. Let your body's instincts and feedback guide you. And I promise you will THRIVE!

Please note that fasting (intermittent and dry) is NOT a replacement for any conventional treatment protocol, medicine or doctor. However, if you do it the right way, it can steer you in the direction of managing most inflammatory diseases. People have fasted away their arthritic pains, and their uric acid and diabetes issues. These are people who have gone through these conditions for years, and, just by fasting the right way, have noticed an improvement in their conditions. The stories you come across in this book are from real people. If you are on medication of any sort and use it as a crutch, change your lifestyle and start introducing your body to fasting. It may suit you or it may not. But it is worth a try.

This book is dedicated to every human being in the world with the love and hope that they may understand the miracle of life. The intelligence and the immense power of the human body, and its ability to heal and prevent is incredible. Your faith might be shaken and destroyed when death, disease or suffering happens, and we may lose faith in the human body's intelligence and miracles, but I hope that, somehow, we can be inspired to slowly re-align with nature and use the body alongside whatever alternative treatment we choose to prevent and heal.

In no way has this book been written to condemn anyone or any system of medicine, or put down doctors of medicine. It is considered to be 'magic' that we can all use in our lives when it comes to healing, prevention and possibly ways of curing, especially when medicine gives up on disease. Imagine, just imagine, the beauty if it can all work together—medicine when required, and fasting, an integrative, beautiful and powerful prevention and healing system. From cancer to well-being, explore the miracle of dry fasting.

All I want to say is that you lose nothing—absolutely nothing—by trying dry fasting. After all, there is science, and then there are miracles . . .

I dedicate this book to my beloved family, my beautiful girl Tyanna Brooklyn, my wife and the Sangha.

I dedicate these writings to Sheikha Noura Al Nuaimi, who inspired me to use dry fasting with patients across the world and who is no more today but is in a better place. May God bless her soul.

My gratitude to Sheikh Abdulaziz Bin Ali Bin Rashed Al Nuaimi—the Green Sheikh—for the inspiration I have gained from our deep conversations on health, the human body and the mind. In the words of the Green Sheikh, 'We must aim to make food our medicine and not medicine our food. One word you can change the world with is "fast". Another word is "smile". Fasting helps us adjust to as little food as possible while having a very normal life. It is highly recommended for the cleaning of the soul and the heart. It helps us get rid of the restrictions that desires impose on us. Fasting cleanses the body of toxins that accumulate from the food and drink we consume, and is a deeply spiritual practice that is meant to benefit us in body, mind and heart.'

I wish each of you good luck, good health and loads of love.

INTRODUCTION

By the Green Sheikh

Fasting is designed to stimulate your 'mind', empower your 'body' and nourish your 'soul'.

It is an honour for me to co-author and share my reflections on *The Dry Fasting Miracle* with Luke Coutinho. The book is an inspirational guide to the ancient, religious and traditional dry-fasting practice, which is based on knowledge, faith, personal beliefs and experiences. This book, in essence, is a miracle for humankind, as it has the ability to transform people into better, healthier versions of themselves. It teaches them to actually live, and not just survive.

A few years ago, I met Luke as he was helping my elder sister, Sheikha Noura Al Nuaimi, treat her medical condition. Unfortunately, the condition she had eventually took over her body and she succumbed to the illness a few months later, but I saw in Luke a compassionate practitioner who listened to his patients and their experiences, and imbibed them into his own understanding of the body and its workings.

He has a symbiotic relationship of learning and sharing with the people he works with. Obviously, the ultimate aim is healing—what it means and how to achieve it. In this book, he has shared what he experienced and learnt while looking after my sister.

Healing comes in different forms—whether medical, spiritual, emotional or traditional.

One of the things my sister tried out during the healing process was dry fasting. This struck Luke, as he was inspired by the notion of fasting and how this one practice could bring a nation together. As my sister and I shared the same beliefs and practices, I felt it would be an immense joy to spread this knowledge that I learnt through faith to others.

Dry fasting

Fasting is a way to please and be obedient to God. In ancient times, people fasted to worship, to sacrifice, to heal and to sustain well-being. The essence of fasting can be summed up in a few words—refraining from all food, drink and sexual activity, commencing at dawn and ending at dusk.

Fasting is the fourth of the five pillars of the Islamic faith. Fasting is participating in the abstinence (*sawm*, or *syam*) that takes place in the holy month of Ramadan, which occurs in the ninth Islamic month. It is a remarkable display of communal worship that is characterized not only by a heightened sense of piety but also by a greater emphasis laid upon family and social ties.

The wisdom behind fasting is that it is an act of worship performed for Allah (God), through which the servant (worshipper) draws closer to His Lord by abandoning the things that he loves and desires. In the Quran, Allah (God) says, 'Believers, fasting has been prescribed for you, just as it was prescribed for those before you, so that you may guard yourselves against evil' (The Holy Quran 2:183).

The fast applies to the daylight hours, in which Muslims refrain from eating, drinking, smoking and sexual intercourse with partners. But why does fasting take place only during the day? Allow me to explain. It is during the day that we consume most of our daily intake of food. In fact, during the day, we are mostly engaged in activities that require a lot of energy. At night we rest, allowing our bodies to take a break from the exhaustion of the day. It's been proven that the activities and movements of the body while fasting during daytime lead to the creation of glucose in the body, which is then stored as energy to fuel organs and their functions while increasing metabolism and cleansing the body of toxins.

Breaking the fast

It is recommended that one break the Islamic fast with fruits such as dates, a tradition that goes back to the days of the Prophet. Dates are easily digestible and help to rapidly energize the whole body, making them a rich source of energy and nutrients. Additionally, dates can regulate glucose levels in the body after a long and tiring day of fasting. Even when not fasting, consumption of a few dates before meals will help temper the hunger, which, in turn, will help curb overeating.

Further fasting days

There are days on which fasting is prohibited—those that coincide with Eid al-Fitr and Eid al-Adha. These are the two main annual Islamic celebrations. Eid al-Fitr is the festival of breaking the fast and happens immediately after Ramadan, and Eid al-Adha (also known as the Greater Eid) is the second celebration of the year and is the festival of sacrifice.

During Ramadan, where fasting is obligatory, you're allowed to break your fast under certain circumstances. Those exempt from fasting are the sick, the elderly, travellers and women who are pregnant, menstruating or lactating. This group is allowed to observe fasting but discontinue, and then compensate for it with an equal number of fasting days later in the year. However, should they be physically unable to do so, they are obliged to feed a needy person for each day that they have missed their fasting.

Types of dry fasting

There are different types of fasting in Islam. They are:

1. Fasting as a duty during Ramadan.
2. Making up for the fasts missed during Ramadan.

3. Voluntary fasting. Normally observed on Mondays and Thursdays, such fasting can occur weekly, monthly or annually. These can either be practised on consecutive days following the month of Ramadan or on any chosen six days during the month proceeding Ramadan.
4. Another type of voluntary fasting entails three days of fasting a month, starting on the night a full moon is seen, known as the white days—the thirteenth, fourteenth and fifteenth days of the Arabic or the Hijiri calendar. Those who want a challenge can alternate the days of fasting for the whole year—one day of fasting, followed by one day of non-fasting. The best example of fasting is that by King David (Prophet Dawood), who used to fast one day and eat on the next.

Three stages of Ramadan

The month of Ramadan can be divided into three parts, each signifying a teaching from God. The first reflects the Mercy of Allah (Rehmah); the second reflects the Forgiveness of Allah (Maghfirah); and the third reflects the Safety from Hell (Nijat). The Holy Prophet Muhammad said: 'It [Ramadan] is the month whose beginning is mercy, middle is forgiveness and end emancipation from the fire [of hell].'

Fasting and family

Family unity or togetherness during Ramadan is an important aspect of fasting. During this month, the whole family gathers around the table or dines with the food being placed on the floor lined up on a traditional dining carpet, or a *mufarash*, to break their fast. This strengthens family ties while sharing joy and happiness with each other. Historically, in various cultures around the world, mealtimes would be when everyone would get together. Due to our modern routines and busy schedules, the family may not always be able to get together and enjoy a meal, but Ramadan is the perfect time for the family to come together for *suhoor* (a late or a last meal before the start of the fast) and iftar (the first meal after completion of the daily fast together). Therefore, Ramadan encourages the family to break the fast together every day of the month. At these times, when eating together as a family, we remember Allah's blessings and inspire each other to have a more productive Ramadan. This fosters the positive feelings of belonging and togetherness.

Fasting and children

One of the most important teachings we pass down to our children is fasting, raising them to practise it for an entire month, or part of it, or even a few days, once a year, to keep their faith intact and their traditions alive. Teaching them the intellectual, physical and spiritual aspects of it is the duty of parents. Children can start fasting from the age of five, and are motivated using challenges and rewards in the form of gifts or things they like to play with. It's not necessary for children to fast for the whole cycle of thirty days or completely refrain from food and water—a few hours will suffice—but then gradually, with their parents' guidance, they start fasting for longer hours or more days until they come of age.

Fasting and behaviour change

When our digestive system is at rest, our mind, too, is at rest. So fasting during Ramadan is a great catalyst for change—for life improvement, for changing undesirable behaviour or habits that would normally be challenging at any other time. As there is abstinence from dusk till dawn for a month, it presents a great opportunity for one to change for the better and adopt healthier lifestyle techniques.

Patience is the key to fasting. In Arabic, 'patience' is described as imprisoning or preventing desire. Therefore, fasting is the practice of patience—theoretically, physically and spiritually.

Fasting and social healing

Fasting can heal and solve many individual, family and socio-national challenges. It is a tradition in many religious and spiritual practices, and has seeped into wellness circles as a therapeutic means to a new lifestyle. It is not just an individual practice but allows those practising it to know and respect each other while creating harmony, solidarity and a sense of community. Fasting in the light of worship is purification of the soul and the heart while simultaneously dissolving all racial differences, removing hatred, avoiding conflict and eliminating lustful desires and greed. Fasting improves relationships and helps heal both psychologically and socially; it helps to avoid anger and violence. The most sincere mode of fasting is associated with contentment, fulfilment, patience and kindness. And, as the Prophet said, 'Contentment is a treasure that is never exhausted.'

Fasting and social responsibilities

Fasting is centred on acknowledging and supporting the hungry, the poor and the less fortunate in society. It involves taking care of neighbours and helping strangers or visitors in need, with whom we can share not only food but also love and respect. A noble person, when he breaks his fast, can do so by eating with the poor in his neighbourhood, creating strong bonds of love and harmony and preventing envy and hatred seeping into hearts. Ultimate happiness is rooted in relationships and the act of giving. Many people from different social classes gather to break their fast together during Ramadan, eating the same food on the same table, creating a sense of unity and equality. A wise man was once asked what other reason could be offered for fasting, and this was his response, 'So the wealthy can feel and taste hunger as experienced by the poor and not forget about them.'

Fasting and sustainability

Every year more than 1.65 billion people around the world celebrate Ramadan. A few years ago, I wrote an

Arabic article titled 'Adaat wa Ibadaat', which in English means 'Habits and Rituals'.

It focused on our daily habits of consumption and lifestyle during the holy month, taking its principle message from the Quran—'Eat and drink but waste not by excess, for God loves not the wasters' and 'Be not excessive! Indeed, He does not like those who commit excess' (The Holy Quran 7:31).

During Ramadan, the Al Ihsan Charity Association based in Ajman provided more than 100,000 iftar meals every day of the month to fifteen locations around mosques and labour camps in Ajman and Ras Al Khaimah, along with smaller towns and cities. This included the staples of rice, flour, cooking oil and dry fruits or fresh meat, distributed to more than 15,000 families and children of all nationalities.

In 2019, more than 50,000 volunteers in eight countries (the UAE, Oman, Bahrain, Kuwait, Saudi Arabia, Jordan, Bosnia and Egypt) prepared to distribute 1,000,000 snack boxes through a social-responsibility campaign run annually during the holy month, called Ramadan Aman. The snack boxes each contained seven pieces of dates, a cupcake and water, and were distributed to all those found driving on the roads just fifteen minutes before the breaking of their fast, to avoid the risk of them speeding home and thereby averting accidents. There are more than thirty well-organized charities in the UAE that are doing something that is both similar and different, collaborating as well as competing with each other, with their main focus on charitable causes and on serving humanity.

During my research through the years, I have tried to find statistics for waste generation in the UAE during Ramadan, but found no actual figures. Recently, it was mentioned in the local media that 600 tonnes of food, or maybe even more, are thrown away every year in the UAE, but I am not quite convinced about this! In reality, a majority of people donate regularly to charities and share food with low-income groups in need. Of course, there are those who are wasteful, but we can always set examples for them. We can think before we act, live in moderation and eat better and healthier local food that promotes sustainable living (dates and water or yoghurt, and organic food). If we closely monitor our daily habits, we can make small changes that will result in huge differences; we can not only prevent wastage but even health problems such as obesity and diabetes.

A few examples: Go shopping after, and not before, breaking your fast. Buy what you need and not what you desire. Decide on how many hours you need to cook and whether you are going to share the food with others. Education, awareness and attitude towards consumption is the most catalytic agent to making a small, simple act have a huge impact on our daily lives and on our environment. It is the blessing, or 'barakah' of Ramadan to be thankful and appreciative of the real wealth in our lives. God has given us the honour, or 'amanah', to be more conscious of the environment and its resources, to be wise about our social and environmental responsibilities, and to be compassionate towards other living creatures.

My fasting philosophy

My fasting experience is based on what a wise man once said: 'Any man or woman can fast, but it is only the wise who knows how to break the fast.' My first attempt at fasting during Ramadan was at the age of six, where I succeeded in lasting till dusk. I went on till dusk on some days but on others, my young body couldn't handle it. The following years I patiently waited for Ramadan so I could complete my challenge; I was only able to fast for a full month at the age of nine. Now I hardly miss a day unless I feel ill or am out on an international trip. To this day, I fast the whole month either for twenty-nine or thirty days (depending on the lunar calendar) and voluntarily follow the six days of the month after Ramadan, called Shawwal. One day of Ramadan is equal to ten normal non-fasting days, so six days of fasting is equal to sixty days. So the total would be 360 days, and the lunar calendar is less than the solar calendar by eleven days.

My lifestyle during Ramadan tends to be more disciplined, healthy and centred on quality time with family and loved ones. I usually break the fast with the whole family, and sometimes with friends, starting with three or seven dates, leben (butter milk) and then some traditional Emirati meal such as harees, threed, machbous or biryani, washed down with authentic Ramadan juices and ending with delicious Arabic delights or rice puddings containing zafran and pistachio. Following our meal, we perform our night prayers and end the day with a light meal after midnight, called suhoor. We get a little sleep before waking up again for the *fajir* (the first prayer at dawn), and then sleep for another few hours. Office starts at 9 a.m. and ends at 2 p.m., by which time I am usually on my way home to get a little rest or a short power nap to gather my energy. I then recite the Quran for thirty minutes and spend another thirty to forty minutes doing some light exercise before starting my volunteer work—to help, inspire and motivate other volunteers while assisting them in distributing snack boxes to fasting drivers at traffic intersections. Every day we go to different places in the UAE, and also visit other countries as part of our campaign.

Here, as a metaphor for the concept on fasting, I would like to share my experience of working as an engineer at a liquefied natural gas (LNG) company. In 1992, when I was working as a process engineer at the LNG plant, I experienced entire systemic shutdowns on three occasions. These happened annually for about thirty–thirty-five days during the cooler months in the UAE, along with a few minor shutdowns (for a few weeks). The idea behind these shutdowns was to run an overall systematic maintenance on the company, replace old parts with new ones and initiate malfunction investigation, modification, revamping, troubleshooting and performance tests. All of this was aimed at sustaining the plant operations, improving production streams and enhancing product quality while reducing emissions and effluents. The plant operations and the shutdowns could serve as metaphors for our bodily systems and fasting, and help us see how fasting can prevent bodily malfunction or heal the human ecosystem.

Incidentally, I was voluntarily fasting while writing the major part of this book. The experience was so different—I could see how fasting helped enhance my thought process and forged a deeper connection between mind and body.

So my message to all of you is that eat less—it is far better than eating more—and give dry fasting a chance. It is just waiting to benefit your soul, your body and your emotions.

There's a hidden sweetness
in the stomach's emptiness.

We are lutes, no more, no less.
If the sound box is stuffed
full of anything, no music.

If the brain and the belly
are burning, clean with fasting,
every moment a new song
comes out of the fire.

The fog clears, and a new
energy makes you run up the
steps in front of you.

Be emptier and cry like
reed instruments cry.
Emptier, write secrets with
the reed pens.

When you're full of food and drink,
Satan sits where your
spirit should, an ugly metal
statue in place of the Kaaba.

When you fast, good habits gather
like friends who want to help.

Fasting is Solomon's ring.
Don't give it to some illusion
and lose your power.

But even if you've lost all
will and control, they come
back when you fast,
like soldiers appearing out
of the ground, pennants
flying above them.

A table descends to your
tent, Jesus's table.
Expect to see it, when you
fast, this table spread with
other food better than the
broth of cabbages.

Rumi

1

WHAT IS DRY FASTING?

'All the vitality and all the energy I have comes to me because my body is purified by fasting'

—Mahatma Gandhi

You must always turn to nature when you are sick or afflicted with disease. Nature holds all the answers, and when you align yourself with it, you heal and recover. Dry fasting is one such answer. Dry fasting is complete abstinence from food and water for a particular window during the day, followed by breaking the fast in a specific manner. This window during which one fasts is called the elimination phase, and the window during which one eats is called the building phase.

Dry fasting—or absolute fasting or Hebrew fasting—comes naturally to animals that are sick and wounded. They retire to a secluded place and fast until the body is restored to normal. It's their natural instinct to refuse food during this time of recovery. At the most, they partake only of water and medicinal herbs. Ever seen a sick cat eat grass? The body is intelligent enough to heal. When the crisis is over, the appetite returns naturally. Humans also have fasting instincts, just like animals. But, unfortunately, when we fall sick, in most cases we fail to follow nature. We continue to eat food, even if in small amounts, and suffer because of it.

Go back a thousand years. What did the early man do? Since food was scarce, they could only feast when they hunted—otherwise they fasted. This evolutionary adaptation has made our bodies efficient at fasting even in this era. If one observes children carefully—and even adults, for that matter—the moment they get sick or hurt, their appetite is what drops first. By switching on its healing mechanism, the body uses its natural intelligence to protect us. The appetite is lost for healing to take place as the immune system requires a lot of energy.

One of my clients, Neha Gupta, wrote to me saying that she had completed seventeen hours of fasting yesterday and thirteen-and-a-half hours today. She said she could never have imagined that she could dry-fast and that, too, with no hunger pangs, as she is known in her family as someone with no control over her appetite. She feels calmer now and more composed, with clarity of thought, but, most importantly, she says she feels happy!

The body is made up of five elements: Earth, Water, Fire, Air and Ether. Fasting cleanses the element of Ether. During dry fasting, all vital forces are engaged in cleansing the body. It should be understood that the fast in itself does not bring about a new vital force but removes toxins in the body, which are the real cause of ill health. In the case of a disease, however, dry fasting is most beneficial when one practises it right from the initial stage.

Well, this is just the beginning of what dry fasting does. Read on to know more about the ancient wisdom behind the practice.

2

TYPES OF DRY FASTING

One of my clients, who is a working woman in her thirties and has just started practising dry fasting, wrote to me saying that she gives her body the best of rest and fasting. And the best thing that she says has happened to her is that she doesn't feel sleepy during the day at all. She is more alert than usual and doesn't feel the need for tea, coffee, food or water. She is able to meditate better while on a dry fast. She also feels it has cleared up her brain fog and hopes to incorporate dry fasting and meditation as daily habits in her life.

Let us find out more about dry fasting. There are two types—soft dry fasting and hard dry fasting.

1. Soft dry fasting

This allows an individual to come in contact with water, which could be through washing hands or the face, or bathing. This is preferred for beginners and those who go to office. I recommend you begin with this if you are a working professional and new to dry fasting. Once you get used to this, you may try hard dry fasting, which is on a more advanced level.

2. Hard dry fasting

Hard dry fasting doesn't allow any contact with water, not even while washing clothes, bathing or brushing. When one dry-fasts, the body becomes like a sponge and the skin becomes highly capable of absorbing any moisture that it comes in contact with (even atmospheric moisture).

3

HISTORY OF DRY FASTING

The concept of dry fasting is as old as mankind, perhaps even older. In ancient times, fasting was regarded as a means of purification of the mind and the body. If one reads historical or spiritual texts, there are numerous instances to prove this. Christianity, Judaism, Gnosticism, Islam, Buddhism, Hinduism, and Indian traditions in South and North America all use fasting in some form or the other for purification, penance, mourning, sacrifice and for deepening the spiritual connection with self. Many faiths even prescribe regular fasting to curb gluttony.

In the United States, the groups that are most well known for their fasting traditions are Episcopalians, Roman Catholics, Lutherans and Jews. Many of our biblical forefathers fasted for some reason or another; and ancient Greeks were great believers in fasting, with Hippocrates strongly advocating it. It is said that Aristotle fasted regularly for greater physical and mental efficiency.

Then there were others such as Galen and Avicenna, who recommended fasting to their patients as part of their prescription.

Yogic practices, to, include fasting and date back thousands of years. The ancient healing practice of Ayurveda includes dry fasting as a means of therapy.

Muslims practise dry fasting almost for a month during Ramadan every year. Fasting has a special place in Jainism and Hinduism as well.

Many married women across India, on the festival of Karva Chauth, observe a yearly dry fast from sunrise to moonrise to pray for the safety and longevity of their husbands.

In Judaism, there are two major dry-fast days and four minor ones that are part of the Jewish year, in which they begin fasting before sundown, when it is still light outside, and end after the next sundown, when it is dark outside and three stars can be seen in the sky.

Greek Christians fast for 180–200 days every year, and their main fasting periods are the Nativity Fast (forty days prior to Christmas), Lent (forty-eight days prior to Easter) and the Assumption Fast (fifteen days in August).

Ancient Egyptians used fasting as a monthly purge to cleanse their bodies, as they believed that all illness came from the food they consumed. The ancient Greek philosopher, Herodotus, described them as the 'healthiest of all men'.

In traditional Chinese medicine, dry fasts are prescribed to influence chi (or qi), considered life force. In qigong (also spelt 'chi-gong' and 'chi kung'), dry fasting is used to increase chi and is often performed in conjunction with acupuncture and acupressure.

American author Mark Twain also believed that fasting was one of the best cures for illness and said, 'A little starvation can really do more for the average sick man than can the best medicines and the best doctors.'

Many religions incorporate fasting into their traditions, often under the premise that it brings one closer to god and that it has a purifying function. In India, it is said that the energy of life flows through a system of branching nerve channels in our body, called *nadi*. When we fast and clear our body of food, we help this universal energy flow smoothly through us. In Judaism, during Yom Kippur, and in Christianity, during Lent, abstinence is symbolic of Jesus fasting for forty days in the desert. In Mormon communities, which dry-fast for twenty-four hours, studies find a lower incidence of diabetes. In Islam, Ramadan calls for an entire month of fasting; it is said that Prophet Muhammad even encouraged fasting twice a week.

Where was dry fasting all this time?

Dry fasting is the most overlooked and yet the most valuable means of healing since time immemorial. However, despite it being an ancient practice, we, somewhere down the line, stopped practising this as routine, because today we have vitamins, supplements, fad diets, various exercise regimes and so-called nutritional programmes that we believe will give us quicker and better results. But good health doesn't have to be so complicated and expensive. The simplest thing one can do is use the intelligence and brilliance of the human body, which has an in-built mechanism to detoxify without having to constantly drink green juices and turmeric lattes. Although superfoods do help us stay healthy, we cannot depend on them alone. Hence, it's important to get back to basics, simplify and do what our ancestors did for centuries. Dry fasting is one of the most sought-after and tried-and-tested ways of tapping into the body's power to heal itself.

'I started fasting at 9.30 p.m. and went strong till 11.30 a.m. for fourteen hours. I'm a foodie and it's the ticking clock that reminds me that I haven't eaten. I broke the fast with warm water, followed by dates and almonds. Then had one green apple and, an hour later, lunch—hummus, bread, salad and some meat. Ended with a cup of coffee (an addiction I'm trying to gain control over). I feel good and raring to go.'

—Anonymous

Why fast?

We are made up of trillions of cells and our overall health depends on the individual health of each of these cells. Dry fasting triggers a cleansing process that reaches each of these cells, and thereby tissues, in the body. This is like rectifying health at the cellular level! The purpose of fasting is to give complete rest to the digestive system. In fact, it is only during fasting that the digestive system can get rest, as, ordinarily, because we eat two or three times every day, it has to constantly keep working.

In Ayurveda, our digestive system is referred to as 'jathara', or Agni (fire). The quality of digestion is based on the health and strength of this digestive fire. It is working 24x7 to digest, secrete, absorb, assimilate and excrete. All of these processes account for almost 80 per cent of the body's energy, leaving the rest of the 20 per cent for other bodily functions. When one decides to dry-fast, there is a complete shutdown of the digestive system. All the organs of the body get some much-needed rest and all the saved energy is then directed to healing, detoxification, purification and rejuvenation, all of which cannot be achieved without fasting. Many people mistake fasting for something similar to starvation. Dr Hereward Carrington, a well-known British-born American investigator of psychic phenomena, explains the difference between fasting and starvation: 'Fast begins with giving up food and ends when one feels hungry, and starvation begins with the feeling of hunger and ends with death.'

4

WHY IS DRY FASTING THE MOST SUPERIOR FORM OF CLEANSING?

Dry fasting, or absolute fasting, is considered the most superior form of cleansing for the body and the mind. It's said that a one-day dry fast is as effective as a three-day water fast or a six-day juice fast.

Why is that? What makes it so powerful?

1. Our body makes its own water

You may not be drinking water during the fast but the body tries to make its own 'metabolic water'! How? As a by-product of the fat that is burnt during the fast. When you fast, hydrogen released from the metabolized fat combines with oxygen from the air to produce water. Unlike the water you drink, this metabolic water is of superb quality, produced by the hard work of your own cells. It is almost like it erases all the negative information that was part of the body before the fast, allowing cells to experience a kind of rebirth, taking in moisture from the air and supplying it to the cells. This phenomenon, which is the main healing mechanism of dry fasting, is what sets it apart from all other kinds of fasting.

So even though it is called dry fasting, it is not quite as dry as people would imagine. Water (a certain amount of it) is indeed essential and undertaking long periods of dry fasting is not possible in the absence of this metabolic water. Water is made scarcer, enough to create some healthy competition among cells, causing diseased or otherwise weakened cells to die off. However, in no way is water completely absent.

The myth that man cannot live more than three days without consuming water is untrue, as the longest dry fast on record has been for eighteen days (if at all planning to dry-fast over a long period, please do so with medical supervision). The reason for this is that the body is capable of producing its own water internally in the process of metabolizing fats.

2. It targets and reduces inflammation, and is immunostimulatory

Inflammation and low immunity are the root causes of any disease—be it cancer, cardiovascular problems, diabetes or simply the inability to lose weight. The body cannot have inflammation without water. Pathological bacteria, viruses and other microbes love a wet environment, which is ideal for them to thrive in—shortage of water is like a kill switch for them.

Dry fasting annihilates microbes and eliminates inflammation the same way a swamp gets rid of mosquitoes and other insects when it dries up. Think of this shortage of water as a cleansing drought. It ups competition among the cells of the body, which vie for whatever water is available to them—so, in a sense, it is a real survival-of-the-fittest scenario for the limited metabolic water there is.

'I have been dry-fasting for a few days and have seen some amazing results in my body. And it's great to follow, as I explained to my mom in Kolkata over the phone. She has been dry-fasting for only three to four days but said that the pain in her leg had already gone down by 90 per cent and that there had been a lot of overall improvement in her body. Thank you, Luke, and all members of the Sangha community for guiding and motivating me.'

—Anonymous

3. It enables the burning of toxins as opposed to the flushing out of toxins via urine, bowel movement, kidneys, liver and skin

Dehydrated cells act as furnaces that burn toxic matter, which are basically the diseased, weaker cells, or rogue cells, that lose out in the competition for limited water. Also, the body, during a dry fast, absorbs atmospheric carbon dioxide and nitrogen to manufacture its own amino acids. Since there is no water to flush out these endogenous toxins, these are eliminated through a unique mechanism that is dormant during less rigorous modes of fasting. Each cell, thus, self-combusts, becoming the furnace that burns up its own waste.

'I completed fourteen and fifteen hours of dry fasting on consecutive days. Because of this, I have no UTI now, and easy motions when I wake up. I can feel that my body has detoxified more with dry fasting. Thanks a lot, Sir. You have been such a motivation. Now I'm sure that I can eliminate all UTI-causing bacteria from my body. Feeling awesome that even someone like me can dry-fast. Will practise dry fasting whenever I can. I am sending you prayers, blessings and positivity.'

—Sonaa Rajwar

Only the strongest and healthiest cells survive in the extreme conditions that fasting induces, while cysts and benign tumours dissolve as a result of autolysis, a process by which the body sacrifices its most unhealthy and sick cells for its own survival. This procedure is called autophagy, the act of self-digestion by a cell through the action of enzymes originating within that very cell. This demonstrates that only strong, viable cells survive a dry fast and even a short-term dry fast can serve as a powerful prophylactic against malignant tumours. One of my clients, Yogita Sardessai, wrote to me saying that she had had a bad throat infection that healed without medication with only one day of dry fasting for fourteen hours. Never underestimate the natural healing power of the body, which is only strengthened and enhanced by dry fasting.

4. Dry fasting can help manage the effects of radiation exposure

Dr T.A. Voistovish, a director of healing and fasting retreats, has seen some interesting results while treating victims of nuclear radiation who had been exposed to 400 to 600 roentgens as a result of the Chernobyl disaster (a catastrophic nuclear leak in Ukraine in 1986). All of those who included fasting in the treatment recovered quickly. They fasted for about two weeks and their bodily functions were restored at a DNA level, thereby helping reverse the effects of radiation. Even heritable mutations can be reversed, with nucleic acids, DNA and RNA being restored. Even damaged cells have been seen to divide normally.

Regular fasting can also help restore the protective functions of cells and organs against radiation damage. This is particularly important for those who live or work in settings where they are regularly subjected to radiation or have been exposed to palliative radiation in case of cancer treatment. Dry fasting can be highly effective in healing the side effects of chemotherapy.

The process of fasting improves the mechanisms that expel toxic substances, especially those that interfere with the body's proper functioning—such as radionuclides, nitrates, pesticides, heavy metals and other poisons.

'I dry-fast every Friday for at least twenty hours. How has it helped me? I face slight gastric issues on days that I eat, but on the day of dry fasting— voila!—I don't have the slightest feeling of acidity or any such issues. I feel lighter, more energetic. This is my third dry fast and I am so eager to join the global dry fast. I have lost 4 kg in the past four months by following Luke. I have only been eating home-made food and have avoided junk and sugar. I've been eating only what my grandmother used to feed me when I was young and, of course, I've taken the magic pill of exercise, deep breathing and staying happy and blessed!'

—Srividhya

5

THE DETOXIFICATION PHYSIOLOGY BEHIND DRY FASTING

During a fast, it takes about ten–twelve hours for the liver to use up its sugar reserve. When the cells are finally done with digestion and the stored sugar has been used up, the body starts burning its stored fat and produces ketone bodies. As your body enters into a state of ketosis—a state in which the body starts utilizing its fat reserves for fuel—free hydrogen molecules are released. As mentioned earlier, these hydrogen molecules then bond with the oxygen molecules in the blood and water (H_2O) is formed internally. This is metabolic water. It is estimated that, every day, our body is able to produce more than a litre of metabolized water and this freshly synthesized metabolic water is much purer, as it is free of the toxins found in most of the external water we drink.

Without external water, blood and lymph are purified through a sort of internal filtration process. This renewal takes place only thanks to metabolic water. As a result, by the end of the dry fasting period, two of the body's most important fluids—blood and lymph—are detoxified. Correspondingly, all the tissues of the body through which blood and lymph circulate are purified of external content. Hence, it helps in detoxification. This phenomenon of purification is one of the primary benefits of dry fasting.

During dry fasting, the body has a more powerful immune response and can fight inflammation more actively. All inflammation is fed by water. Take, for example, oedemas that contain pus and lymph. When the body is deprived of an inflow of exogenic water, it uses endogenic water carefully—only to feed healthy cells. Damaged cells, as well as various bacteria, viruses and parasites, suffer from this lack of water and die.

During dry fasting, people may often have fever, which is actually a good indicator that the body is fighting infection. Every cell in the body is turned into a kind of furnace or reactor, and the toxins inside are destroyed. If a cell is too damaged, it is eliminated. The increase in body temperature leads to the creation of a strong immunological response. The concentration of biologically active substances in bodily fluids also increases. These include immunoglobulins and immunocompetent cells. The following happens as a result:

1. The production of interferon (an antibody in response to a pathogen) increases.
2. Antitumour and antiviral activity increases.

3. T-lymphocytes proliferate.
4. Bactericidal capacity and phagocytic activity of neutrophils increase.
5. The cytotoxic effect of lymphocytes increases.
6. The growth of microorganisms and their toxicity decreases.

As this process of detoxification takes place, it makes space in the tissues for new stem cells. Stem cells are then released into the blood in higher volume to occupy this vacated 'space' and to promote the regeneration and rejuvenation processes. Hence, dry fasting has a remarkable effect in promoting stem-cell-based regeneration too.

A Russian doctor of biology, named Y. Romanov, says, 'One of the most significant benefits of fasting is the creation and release of stem cells in the body, which increases even more during a dry fast! Basically, as the intense bodily cleanse is initiated, old, sick, and dead cells are released in massive quantities and eliminated through the urine. As this process takes place, there is now more space for cells to be born, and so stem-cell production shifts from being dormant into a state of active production, and stem cells are released throughout the body in high capacity.'

His research was later backed up by a study done by the University of Southern California. Various experiments then followed that proved that after fasting, the body tripled its production and release of stem cells, an effect that could last several months. These facts taken together make dry fasting a highly effective tool to address acute health issues that are inflammatory and immunity-related, as well as degenerative conditions such as Alzheimer's, Parkinson's disease and cases of cancer.

'I have hardly ever visited doctors or taken pills or fallen sick in my life. But, maybe, due to too many temperature fluctuations where I live, for three–four days, I have been experiencing a tickling in my throat, a sign that I might catch a cold and a fever soon. And that's what happened yesterday. There was severe pain in my throat and a rise in my body temperature. I gargled with warm salt and turmeric water and decided to go on a dry fast from 5 p.m. yesterday. And to my surprise, this morning I woke up with absolutely no throat pain. My body temperature was also normal! OMG! So that's the power of dry fast! I have done six–seven dry fasts earlier but it is only this time that I truly understood and experienced what tremendous power the body has to heal itself.'

—Hetal Sutar

6

WHAT HAPPENS DURING
DRY FASTING?

As the body undergoes dry fasting, what are the changes it experiences? Let us try and understand the different stages of dry fasting.

Stage 1 lasts for the first couple of days of the fast or for about twelve–forty-eight hours from the last meal. This stage is when the body transitions into fasting mode—for many of us this is the most challenging part of the process. This stage is when one starts to feel hunger pangs as regular mealtime routines are skipped. Most first-time fasters start to feel a reduction in their energy levels. These effects can induce a negative mood, irritability and impatience. Since the body goes into power-saving mode, there may be a lowering of the heart rate and blood pressure.

Stage 2 starts around the end of Day 2 and lasts until Day 7. A lot of changes begin to happen during this stage, and there may be noticeable changes in physical appearance as well. By this time, ketosis has begun. One might stop feeling hungry and tired. During stages 1 and 2 of the fast, the body expels toxins and damaged cells via urine or stool.

Stage 3 typically happens between Day 8 and Day 15. This stage includes a dramatic improvement in mood and mental clarity, and is the stage 'seasoned' fasters look forward to the most. The body starts going into 'healing mode'. The healing process begins as the digestive system takes a break from the common stress factors and toxins it had been enduring on a daily basis. As a result, there are fewer free radicals and the oxidative stress decreases. When the cumulative effects of this stage add up, it encourages healthy ageing, and there are fewer health complications. Although this has not been researched enough, the healing process seems to improve health for some.

Stage 4 occurs sometime around Day 16 and continues through the duration of the fast. While there may be some changes moving beyond this juncture, there is a daily balance that starts to set in.

Stage 5 involves breaking the fast. Stage 5 may come sooner or later, depending on the fasting goal. How one chooses to end the fast is critical. Depending on how long the fast has been, one may need to ease his/her way back into eating to avoid discomfort and complications.

'I am amazed at dry fasting . . . and the best part is I'm free from coffee addiction and, best of all, have no cravings . . . Simply too good. Dry fasting is certainly going to be part of my life . . . twice a week for certain!'

—Chandrika Nair

7

BENEFITS OF DRY FASTING: MIND, BODY AND SOUL

Now that we are aware of what the body undergoes during the various stages of dry fasting, let's find out what its benefits are.

Physical benefits

1. Boosts immunity

With the world afflicted with so much disease, each of us must start looking at investing in our immunity. It's the first and last line of defence, including against cancer.

When our digestive system—the main consumer of energy in our body—is at rest, our body diverts all the energy towards repair and regeneration, including the immune system. The immune system gets recharged when the body is fasting. Research suggests that fasting can lead to a reduction in the number of white blood cells, which, in turn, can trigger the immune system to start producing new white blood cells. These new white blood cells (also called lymphocytes) are a key component of our body's immune system.

Studies have shown that prolonged fasting switches off a gene called PKA, which is the key gene that needs to shut down to allow stem-cell regeneration. It's like giving a green signal to stem cells to go ahead and proliferate, leading to a rebuilding of the immune system.

This aspect of dry fasting is hugely beneficial to cancer patients undergoing chemotherapy. While chemotherapy does a lot to save lives, it also causes significant collateral damage to the immune system. Fasting can help mitigate some of the harmful effects of chemotherapy.

'I have had an eye infection with redness and itching for almost two weeks now. I've tried many natural remedies but nothing has worked. I only got temporary relief. I was also given eye drops for a week, but, again, with no results. Last week I decided to dry-fast. The next day the redness in my eye was almost 50 per cent better. It was a dramatic change. Only later did I realize that this was due to the dry fast, as I wasn't on any medication then. Can't wait to do the three-day dry fast.'

—Aruna Anand

2. Keeps inflammation and infection in check

Inflammation occurs only in the presence of water. Where there is no water, there is no inflammation. Since dry fasting means going without food and water, there is a marked improvement in inflammatory markers like CRP (C-reactive protein) and ESR (erythrocyte sedimentation rates). There have been instances in which an absolute fast for three to five days has cured people of lifelong allergic reactions and chronic joint pains. Inflammatory gut issues also get resolved, as fasting cleanses the gastrointestinal tract and renews its mucosal lining.

Shivani, one of my clients, has been following our programme since April 2018. She got her hsCRP (high-sensitivity C-reactive protein) levels tested in December that year and, to her surprise, the readings turned out to be 4.1 mg/dL. The average reading is 1–3 mg/dL. She was surprised as she had already been practising intermittent fasting for several months, and the reading shouldn't have been so high. She continued fasting and got the hsCRP levels checked again in February 2019—they had increased to 5.2 mg/dL. She continued and got tested again in May 2019 and this time the reading had shot up to 10.1 mg/dL. She was confused about why this was happening, as she had been eating mindfully and regularly working out as well. Then she realized it was the stress from her personal issues. She promised herself that she would reduce stress and incorporate both intermittent and dry fasting in her routine, along with regular exercise. She also started eating only raw food until lunch (at least four–five days a week). Her next report said it all. From 10.1 mg/dL in May, her reading had come down to 1.32 mg/dL in September. Her learning is:

Health = what you eat + exercise + your mental and emotional state

Research establishes that fasting leads to a drop in inflammation, especially during Ramadan, which is nothing but a dry fast. Dry fasting helps lower concentrations of inflammatory markers such as CRP, Interleukin-6 (IL-6) and tumour necrosis factor (TNF). The inflammation-lowering effects of dry fasting are more powerful than of intermittent fasting.

Research has shown that fasting reduces the release of monocytes—a type of WBC—into the blood stream. These cells go into 'sleep mode', becoming less capable of initiating an inflammatory response than those found in people who do not fast.

Thus, dry fasting can be beneficial in checking most inflammatory diseases, including weight loss, obesity, diabetes, cardiovascular and autoimmune diseases, inflammatory bowel diseases, brain degenerative conditions—and even cancer.

Additionally, dry fasting is of great help in healing inflamed, painful and stiff joints, such as those experienced in arthritis, gout and rheumatism.

Extended and recurring periods of dry fast have also been known to help people battle yeast and bacterial infections such as thrush (caused by *Candida albicans*), vaginal infections and UTI.

> *'Completed thirty-six hours of dry fasting today and am still feeling so good. I did have a little headache, but that was expected. The main achievement is that the pain in my body and the stiffness have gone away, and my fibromyalgia pain has also been reduced. I am feeling calm and happy.'*
>
> —Yashoda Bela

3. Induces autophagy

Dry fasting triggers a phenomenon called 'autophagy', or 'self-eating'. It's a powerful and inbuilt mechanism in our body, in which it tries to sacrifice its sickest cells. Diseased and worn-out cells are removed, certain cell proteins are broken down and other toxic cells and debris are recycled for energy.

This powerful phenomenon was discovered in 2016 by a Japanese biologist, Yoshinori Ohsumi, who was also awarded the Nobel Prize for this breakthrough research on how cells aged and recycled their content in this process.

4. Improves cardiac health

A 2012 study on Ramadan dry fasting showed a significant improvement over the past ten years in the incidence of heart risk in individuals based on other cardiovascular risk factors, such as lipid profile, blood pressure, weight and waist circumference.

Dry fasting helps lower bad cholesterol, boost good cholesterol and lower inflammation, each of which has a positive effect on cardiovascular health.

A study conducted on thirty people during Ramadan found that:

- In females, there was a significant increase in HDL cholesterol levels.
- In males, there was a significant decrease in weight, total cholesterol and triglycerides.

Another study found that people who dry-fasted for twenty-four hours had a lower risk of coronary heart disease compared to non-fasters.

Fasting purifies blood and lymph, and clears blood vessels of plaque and inflammation. Also, as blood purification takes place, levels of the circulating triglycerides come down, which has been seen to have a positive effect on cholesterol levels.

5. Improves liver health

Fasting heals liver cells, boosts enzymatic activity and checks inflammation. Studies on Ramadan have reported the positive effects fasting has on non-alcoholic fatty liver disease.

6. Improves bone health

Apart from better management of pain and inflammation in case of bone-related conditions, fasting has been found to increase levels of a vital hormone called the

'I have had a bad throat ache and cough since October. I went to two ENTs in India, who made me go through an endoscopy and said it was acid reflux. They put me on medication for acidity. I took it for almost a month and felt only about a 50 per cent relief in cough but the pain was the same; I couldn't even breathe properly as it would get really painful.

After taking up the three-day challenge of intermittent and dry fasting for sixteen–eighteen hours a day, with no gluten and no dairy, I realized that I had no throat ache and that the cough, too, was almost negligible.

I think either gluten or dairy was causing the acid reflux, which then led to the throat ache and the cough.

Now I will only just have to figure out whether it was gluten or dairy.

I want to thank you, Luke, for showing us this holistic way of living.

These past three days my energy levels and sleep quality have been so much better than before.'

—Poonam Dhawan

parathyroid hormone (PTH). This plays a key role in bone formation and density. Thus, a spike in PTH leads to better bone resorption and formation, and an increase in calcium levels.

7. Improves kidney health

A lot of micronutrients such as magnesium and calcium get stored in the bones, which can be used while fasting. A study conducted over five days on food and water deprivation showed a decrease in weight and all measured circumferences, and a considerable improvement in renal function. However, since kidney cases are sensitive and need a personalized approach to treatment, it is of extreme importance that you keep your health professional and doctor in the loop before trying anything out. While some kidney conditions require you to consume large amounts of water (for kidney stones and UTI), some may require you to restrict your water intake (such as in the case of renal failure and dialysis). Customization and expert guidance, therefore, is crucial.

8. Keeps PCOD in check

Fasting has an overall positive effect on polycystic ovary disease (PCOD). However, since hormones are tricky and work in concert with each other, they can be challenging to handle. Studies have shown that short-term fasting helps increase the level of luteinizing hormone (LH) in obese women, which is known to have a positive effect on their ovulatory cycles. Fasting also helps lose weight (studies have shown a 7–10 per cent loss in weight over a period of six–twelve months), which can, in turn, check the symptoms of PCOD and associated insulin sensitivity.

9. Can improve thyroid health

Fasting and its effects on thyroid health is one of the most debated topics in medical circles. While some say that fasting can have a positive effect on it, some say that it can, rather, add to any problems there might already be. This is because of the involvement of hormones, which, as mentioned earlier, can be extremely tricky. However, several studies have shown that fasting doesn't alter the concentration of the thyroid stimulating hormone (TSH) in the body, nor does it need any change in the dosage of thyroid medication in an individual. In case of hypothyroidism, it is not a good idea to fast for an extended period of time. This is because our body can interpret it as a state of starvation, to which it then responds by switching on its flight-or-fight mode to conserve energy and further shut down metabolism. Because of this, it is best for individuals with a thyroid condition to fast for shorter durations. Listen to your body and do what suits you. Individuals with mild to moderate levels of hyperthyroidism can fast safely for shorter durations. Both women and men going though hormonal imbalance may want to keep their health professional in the loop before adopting any kind of fasting routine. It is advisable to first correct any hormonal imbalance and then go on to fasting.

10. Can slow down the process of ageing

Ageing is inevitable. However, thanks to our current lifestyles and overexposure to processed food, lack of sleep, pollution, fad exercise regimes and diet programmes, we age faster today. Our biological age is way more than our chronological age. But fasting can delay the ageing process and be the key to longevity and youthfulness. A study by Harvard researchers have shown that fasting delays ageing by altering the activity of mitochondrial networks inside our cells. This means that fasting can also help us get a better handle on our age-related disorders and diseases. It is said that the regular practice of dry fasting can extend life, youth and vitality by fifteen–twenty-five years.

11. Boosts stem-cell regeneration and, hence, immunity

Science is showing stem-cell therapy to be a promising field for our health and healing but it can get really expensive. But the good news is that dry fasting is a free and non-invasive way to get stem-cell therapy! Each of us are essentially made of stem cells. They are the most primitive form of cells—the very first type in the human body before they start getting differentiated according to function, say the cardiac muscle cell, the brain cell, etc. To put it simply, stem cells are capable of assuming any cell type and function, thereby heightening the body's capacity to heal damage and boost immunity. A newborn has more than 1 stem cell per 10,000 cells, but this number gradually starts to decrease as the body ages. This is precisely why parents think of preserving the stem cells in the umbilical cord of a newborn, so in case the child contracts a disease during his lifetime, these cells can be used to repair and regenerate diseased tissue. When we fast, our body undergoes autophagy and tries to sacrifice its sickest cells. The more the body tries to eliminate these sick and dead cells, the more space is created in the body for more new stem cells. Dry fasting activates the release of these new stem cells from the bone marrow into the blood.

12. Can improve skin health

Most people report an immediate change in the way their skin looks and feels with regular dry fasting. The level of clean-up and detoxification dry fasting induces is bound to reflect on the skin. Other aspects that are triggered during fasting that could change the way our skin feels and looks are:

- Decrease in inflammation and the number of free radicals.
- Regeneration of new skin cells.
- Improvement in gut microflora (the ratio of good to bad bacteria).
- Enhanced insulin sensitivity, which helps manage high blood sugar levels. This is thought to help maintain the levels of the two most important proteins in our

skin—collagen and elastin—that are responsible for giving it structure and elasticity.

Fasting has the most profound effects on skin issues such as acne, eczema, allergies, rashes, pigmentation and dullness.

However, it is important to understand that how and what one eats during the non-fasting window is also crucial. If one is dry-fasting but not eating well—undereating or overeating during the building phase—skin health can actually start deteriorating. It can start to look more dull, aged and wrinkly because it's not getting the right nutrients. When we enter the eating window, our cells become like sponges waiting to receive nutrition. If we try to 'diet' during this phase, we deprive our cells of nutrients they need to function. This can be dangerous. Hence it's necessary to know how to eat right during the feeding phase. Stick to simple staples and fresh home-made food, such as dal and rice, khichdi and soup. Avoid any fried or hard-to-digest food, because that could overwhelm the digestive system.

It's important to respect both the phases of fasting to experience a positive effect on skin health. In cases where one is eating right in the building phase, the effects can be miraculous. In one of the global dry fasting challenges we rolled out, a lady who was a regular faster experienced her dead skin peeling away while new skin began growing in its place. This is more likely with prolonged hours of fasting.

13. Improves the functioning of the digestive system

Dry fasting allows the overworked stomach to rest. It helps cleanse the gastrointestinal tract and rids the body of all toxic matter. It also renews mucosal linings and promotes good bacteria in the gut. Dry fasting benefits individuals who complain of bloating, flatulence, indigestion, leaky gut and constipation. If dry fasting is done the right way, it can also provide relief from more complex digestive disorders such as irritable bowel syndrome, gastritis, peptic ulcers and *H. pylori* infections. When a person fasts, hydrochloric acid secretion automatically reduces and this paves the way for healing. Usually, there's a reduction in pain, bloating and discomfort of any sort. If there is any pain because of peptic ulcers during fasting, one can tackle it by alternate hot and cold compress (five minutes each) using a large flannel cloth across the midsection.

14. Can help fight, and even prevent, cancer

We often blame bad genes for cancer, but only three–four kinds of cancer are truly genetic and there is little we can do about it. But for the rest of the kinds of cancer, there is a lot we can do. The world today has almost accepted the fact that thyroid medications are for life, diabetes is irreversible, and cancer is bad luck and the end of life. We need to understand that our mindsets have been moulded today.

Do you not see and hear stories of people reversing cancer and diabetes? Are you aware of cases where people have safely weaned off their thyroid medication by correcting their lifestyle? There wasn't any magic pill or magic diet involved there. They just realized that they got sick because of a faulty lifestyle and worked towards correcting that to see if their body would respond. And it did.

As mentioned earlier, fasting helps trigger autophagy and this phenomenon can be instrumental in cancer management. It helps boost immunity and protect normal and healthy cells from the toxic effects of anti-cancer agents such as chemotherapy drugs.

Studies have reported that dry fasting can help reduce the side effects of chemotherapy, radiotherapy and targeted drug therapy. Cancer patients who do fast tend to have higher tolerance to chemotherapy, fewer side effects and higher energy levels as compared to those who don't.

According to a study, an overnight fast of more than thirteen hours can reduce the risk of early-stage breast cancer. Dry fasting has the capacity to heal and block the progression of cancer and even destroy tumours. Cancerous cells are nothing but our own body cells that start mutating and need carbohydrates as energy to multiply, but when we dry-fast, our body utilizes energy obtained from the metabolism of fat cells; as a result, cancerous cells are not able to multiply and there is autolysis and reduction in abscesses, tumours and cysts too.

'My first experience with dry fasting for three days was a breeze; this surprised me, as I had problems with my digestive system prior to dry fasting and I am the kind of person who cannot have a meal late, forget about skipping one altogether. It always leads to headaches and gastric issues! I was used to having three cups of tea a day.

But here comes the best part:

1. After only three days of dry fasting, I do not feel like having three cups of tea. It is down to one.
2. I don't feel so hungry any more—there are no hunger pangs.
3. Gastric issues are less.
4. No acid reflux.
5. I feel lighter.
6. I do not feel like having dinner at all.'

—Charanpreet

Prolonged fasting also lowers levels of IGF-1, a growth-factor hormone that has been linked to ageing, tumour progression and cancer risk.

Often during treatment, when the cancer gets worse, dry fasting can help confuse the cancer cells by creating extreme environments in the body that only normal cells can quickly respond to.

15. May make chemotherapy more efficient

Most people see chemotherapy in a negative light—and for good reason, especially when we are explained the toxic side effects of it and the fact that it does not guarantee a cure. But now that you have decided to go for it, there's no point wasting time in seeing the bad in it. Instead, channel that energy into what you can do, how the side effects can be managed, how the healthy cells can be saved and how one can improve the efficacy of chemotherapy.

So what can you actually do about this? Try short-term fasting. In other words, fasting according to our biological clock, which simply means eating an early dinner (close to sunset) and breaking it by sunrise—that is, sunset-to-sunrise fasting (explained later in the book).

There is clinical scientific evidence showing how smart fasting can achieve a reduction in side effects and improve the efficacy of chemotherapy. The biological clock controls almost every function in the human body. Over the past year, we saw hundreds of patients who fasted as per their biological clock and saw little or no side effects of chemotherapy; plus they came out of it much stronger and the doctors were happy with their blood counts and the fact that no chemotherapy cycle was skipped because of low immunity, poor blood count or weakness. Clinical medicine is also leaning towards smart fasting playing a role in reducing the chances of a recurrence in cancer.

However, please make an informed decision when you opt to dry-fast during chemotherapy. What we have seen in our cancer patients has been nothing short of phenomenal. We encouraged our patients to finish dinner at sunset and then maintain an easy twelve-hour fast until morning; we allowed them to drink plain water during the fast. Patients reported not feeling hungry in twelve hours and chose to continue for thirteen and even fifteen hours comfortably, post which they broke their fast with fruit and a wholesome breakfast.

What did they experience?

- Better and deeper sleep.
- Little or no nausea.
- Little to no constipation/diarrhoea.
- Little or no hair fall.
- Less pigmentation of skin.
- More energy levels (many resumed work immediately!).
- A loss of fear for the upcoming chemo cycles because of how good they were feeling.
- Loss of cravings for caffeine, sugar and carbohydrates.

Well, it's simple science.

The human body is not designed to break down and digest late dinners and heavy meals. It is too much stress on the system. In the fasting state, the body directs energy towards building, repair, rejuvenation, immune function, clean-up and detoxification. The sooner you get the toxins out of your body, the better it's going to be for the patient and the body. Our body has its own intelligent detox mechanism that gets activated when one is fasting.

A few things to keep in mind if you are trying this:

- Please listen to your body. The first two–three days will be a little uncomfortable. Chances are that you may feel hungry but that's purely out of habit. Once you get through these two–three days, it will be a breeze and you will feel amazing.
- Listen to your body always. If you need to take medicines, take them at the time your doctor has asked you to, and make sure you eat—don't take it on an empty stomach. Or work with your doctor to adjust the medication outside of your fasting window.
- The circadian-rhythm fasting is not a game or a competition. Listen to your body and break the fast when your body tells you to. You may get nine hours of fast the first day, then eleven hours, and then twelve. Build it up one day at a time. Don't prolong the fast more than required, as your body also needs nutrients to build you, protect you and provide energy to fight the cancer.
- This fast can be practised by people without cancer too, and is a powerful way to invest in prevention and recovery.
- Please refrain from late dinners and work towards a lifestyle that includes early dinners. This lifestyle habit will sort out most health issues, especially if you have cancer and are undergoing chemotherapy.

- Most importantly, work on your mindset! Since you are going through chemotherapy, it's best to change your mindset too. While the chemotherapy is going on, visualize and believe that it's only doing good for you. Visualize that it's entering your system, killing the cancer cells, and making you healthier and stronger.

You lose nothing by trying.

'Thank you for showing a systematic way of dry-fasting. Whoever told me I had to eat every two hours because I was diabetic has been proved wrong. I have taken no diabetes medication for the past three-and-a-half months, and I feel good. In my eating phase, I have water, dates, soaked nuts and fruits, and for dinner regular food, before starting my fast. Yes, walking does matter. The day before yesterday, I managed to walk 6000 steps. Visualization and affirmation also helped me. I followed the left nasal breathing at bedtime. Like you suggested, I take apple cider vinegar before meals and chew my food well. And, most importantly, I try not to allow stress to get to me. I just laugh and divert my thoughts, telling myself that it's not good for me—don't take this gift, return it, throw it! And it works! I feel light and move on to other thoughts. Small things lead to a big change.'

—Tejal

16. Keeps diabetes in check

When it comes to diabetes, discussions and solutions often revolve around fasting and postprandial sugar levels. Hardly do we talk about the health of the pancreas. As noted earlier, during dry fasting, ketone bodies are formed and there is regeneration of damaged pancreatic cells, thus increasing insulin sensitivity. Dry fasting, coupled with a tailor-made food plan, is one of the most natural ways to manage or possibly reverse diabetes. So many diabetics who practise dry fasting regularly measure their blood sugar levels and if they see it going too low, break the fast.

17. Helps tackle autoimmune diseases

Autoimmunity starts at the gut. Today we live in a world where food is accessible 24x7. We eat and drink continuously and never give the digestive system any chance to rest or repair. The sensitive gut lining is often damaged due to lifestyle issues and there is slow corrosion of the inner walls of the stomach. When the wall of the gut lining gets damaged, it allows protein molecules from the food we eat to seep into our bloodstream. This causes our immune system to flare up and launch an attack—this is called autoimmunity. Dry fasting is extremely beneficial for all autoimmune and gut-related disorders, because the period spent not eating gives time to the gut lining to repair itself and seal any holes. However, care should be taken that it is not done for a prolonged time, as this would lead to accumulation of ketone bodies, which need to be eliminated. Hence, a dry fast of sixteen hours, three days a week, is recommended more than prolonged fasting.

18. Aids weight loss, mostly at the expense of fat

It's obvious that you will lose weight during a dry fast. You may lose anywhere between 1-3 kg during a three-day fast. However, the weight lost can be a combination of water weight, muscle mass and fat. One must not depend on dry fasting to lose weight. Rather, one must focus on lifestyle changes for sustainable weight management. But if you find your weight loss has hit a plateau, dry fasting can be a powerful way to break that. Dry fasting shocks the body with an extreme change in the eating pattern, and that's what compels it to go into a regulatory mechanism and bring about a response.

While on the one hand, the prospect of losing weight may excite some, on the other, it may worry some others who are aiming to build muscle or are already thin. There is nothing to worry about, though. Dry fasting does not result in significant loss of muscle mass and is, therefore, the best way to treat obesity. If you are already of a slender frame, you can still dry-fast, as most of the weight is regained once you return to normal food. Following a balanced diet after the fast can help in maintaining weight.

Multiple studies have reported a definite loss in weight and fat percentage with Ramadan fasts, especially in case of overweight and obese individuals. However, these effects are modest and short-lived, since most people tend to gain the weight back afterwards, once Ramadan is over. This is only because they change their eating patterns for that particular month and resume all the old habits once Ramadan is over.

Thus, fasting, in no way, should be considered a short cut to lose weight. Weight loss is a great side effect of fasting and will happen anyway because of time-restricted eating. Instead, one must use fasting as a tool to bring discipline into our life. Once this is attained, there will be true and sustained fat loss. Fasting helps reduce cravings, and lowers appetite and hunger—all of which reflect on weight.

So don't jump into dry fasting if you only want to lose weight. You will, but you will also gain all the lost weight, and more if you don't change your lifestyle and your habits.

We receive long mails from people complaining about not even losing an inch while fasting. Well, to being with, change your mindset and intention.

19. Can extend life and youth

Due to its effect on stem-cell production, regular dry fasting can extend life, youth and vitality by fifteen–twenty-five years. Dry fasting has an incredible rejuvenating effect, since it forces the body to eliminate weak and damaged cells that cannot withstand extreme conditions. Cells become stronger and, correspondingly, result in 'healthy offspring' when they divide. Skin, hair and nails glow with health and youth. Acne disappears. Skin gains radiance. Fasting for prolonged periods can also lead to the peeling away of old skin and the generation of new skin.

'I have been following intermittent and dry fasting, depending on the weather conditions, for the past eight months. I am doing it for eighteen–twenty hours once a week, and I have seen amazing results. I have high energy and my concentration level has also improved.

There has also been a huge improvement in my eyesight. I have been wearing spectacles for more than ten years now for nearsightedness, but since I started fasting, I can see read without spectacles. In fact, I have stopped using spectacles for the past seven months. Not just that, my hair loss has also stopped completely and there is a significant improvement in the texture of my skin.'

—Dr Manoti Talwalkar

20. It can heighten taste

As toxins get eliminated from the body, the digestive system and the tongue, there's a heightened sense of smell and taste. This is a remarkable result of dry fasting.

Cleansing of the system leads to a better functioning of the taste buds and to heightened perception. So with fasting, your food will taste better too.

21. Induces higher energy levels

As toxins are removed, one experiences improved energy and vigour. In fact, higher energy levels is one of the most noticeable changes after fasting the right way. As cells clean up their toxic waste, as the digestive system is put to rest, energy levels surge.

'Hello, dear readers, I have broken my dry fast after forty-four hours and I'm full of energy. I ran 10 km both days. I feel so calm and relaxed during the fasting—there's no hunger pangs, no thirst—it's the first time that I have enjoyed so much calm in my body. I love it.'

—Poonam

22. Helps curb appetite

Dry fasting is helpful in regulating the secretion of leptin (satiety hormone) and ghrelin (hunger hormone), and hence can help get appetite in control. Sanchita, one of my clients, has been practising dry fasting almost every day. She eats her dinner at 5 p.m. and is done for the day. She does not chew or eat anything else after that.

She next has breakfast at noon. She actually fasts for nineteen hours. Interestingly, she doesn't feel hungry in between but sometimes tends to break her fast before noon just for a change in routine.

23. Promotes lean muscle growth

Fasting—if done with due respect to both the fasting and the building phases—can prove to be a great tool for body transformation and lean muscle growth.

Many studies have shown that fasting is a great stimulus for the production of the human growth hormone (HGH), which, along with being responsible for proper growth in kids, also contributes to lean muscle growth and recovery, immunity and mitochondrial function. Dry fasting produces more than five times the HGH secreted during intermittent fasting. Yes, there are quick fixes such as injections and supplements for HGH, but that can harm the kidney and the liver. Our body naturally has the ability to do that when it is fasting—this is the beauty and intelligence of the human body, that it can do everything needed to prevent disease, and possibly help you heal and live a long and healthy life. We do not have to look outside of us at all. It's all within us and all we need to do is tap into this intelligence.

Fasting, if practised in synergy with proper exercise, also helps improve overall body mass composition, boost muscle growth and help muscle recovery. A study on fasting conducted among fifteen healthy football players showed higher levels of good cholesterol and a reduction in bad cholesterol and inflammatory markers.

According to Dr Mark Mattson, a professor of neuroscience at Johns Hopkins University, a bodybuilder needs two things to gain muscle definition—training to build muscle and a low fat percentage. To attain this, bodybuilders skip breakfast, work out midday or after a minimum of sixteen hours of fast and then enter the building phase. This way they are able to maintain and build muscle while losing more fat. So contrary to what most people believe, fasting can actually help maintain and build lean muscle. If you are noticing a loss in muscle mass and body tone, then you may not be fasting the right way. Reduce your fasting period and increase your calorie intake during the building phase.

It is not about fasting for sixteen or eighteen hours— it is about reaching the fasting hours that works best for you. A 16:8 fasting-to-eating window has become a new term in society these days.

24. Helps keep asthma in check

Asthma is typically an allergic reaction born of an obstruction in our respiratory passage due to excess mucous accumulation and inflammation, which leads to difficulty in breathing normally.

Mucous is normal and has a protective function. It is, in fact, part of the body's defence mechanism to protect us from invading pathogens, allergens and pollutants by trapping it. However, excess mucous secretion can end up obstructing our respiratory passage.

Since dry fasting reduces inflammation, as is seen in the reduction in CRP levels in a blood report, it can help prevent mucous production, making breathing easier by clearing up the respiratory passages.

'I suffered from allergic rhinitis for more three years. My doctors gave me a combination of drugs to manage my symptoms and also told me that there was no cure for it. But I have been trying out dry fasting for the past two weeks, and, while I still do have continuous sneezing, it doesn't go beyond that. And I haven't had to take a single pill.

I realize there's a lot I have to rectify in my system, and this is just the beginning . . .'

—Prachi Sharma

25. It does not cause dehydration

Can our body undergo dehydration while dry fasting? Not really. Our body produces a hormone called the anti-diuretic hormone (ADH), which, while fasting, gets pushed into the bloodstream and to our kidneys to help regulate the water depletion by absorbing the water we need to keep functioning. So even if we aren't consuming any water or food to hydrate the body, AHD makes sure we have enough water in our blood and other organs to continue all bodily functions properly. Our body is smart enough to know when to produce that hormone, so we do not experience dehydration.

A study in Malaysia found that the total water content in the body remained the same before and after fasting, despite water restriction. Thanks to the release of ADH, the body can compensate for the lack of water by minimizing water loss through lesser urination, thereby creating an internal balance.

Mental benefits

1. Improves brain health

Fasting enhances neurological function. It halts inflammation, ageing and the formation of free radicals. Each of these aspects can have neuro-protective properties on our brain health.

Research by Mark Mattson, head of the laboratory of neurosciences at Johns Hopkins University, has shown that fasting for a couple of days can protect brain function, preventing and possibly managing diseases such as Alzheimer's and Parkinson's. It can boost memory, learning capacity and mood.

Another way dry fasting protects brain health is by producing ketone bodies, which help reduce the amount of 'glutamate'—thought to be a toxin that causes neuronal death. Ketone bodies also help reduce and manage oxidative stress—one of the core reasons why we age.

Research also shows that fasting helps increase the concentration of a growth factor called the brain-derived neurotrophic factor (BNDF), which helps in maintaining memory, cognition, learning capacity, formation of new neural connections (neurogenesis) and neural lifespan.

Even a short-term dry fast can improve brain function by killing harmful or unnecessary cells through autophagy. Through regular episodes of dry fasting, one can experience improved cognition, concentration and creativity, and reduced brain fog, stress and inflammation.

2. Reduces cravings

One of the main reasons we experience cravings is because of toxins. A toxic body always craves sugar and salt, because that is what toxins (or harmful bacteria in the gut) need to thrive. During a fast, when there is complete abstinence from food and water—and the resulting lack of what supports their growth—these bad bacteria perish. The cleaner the body, the lesser the cravings. Many people who fast experience reduced cravings for their age-old habitual food and drink, such as early-morning tea, post-meal dessert and junk food.

During a dry fast, it's natural to experience a loss of psychological hunger. For example, if a person practises dry fasting, psychological hunger will pass in a day. Hence, most people who practise dry fasting say it is easier to endure than water fasting, as hunger pangs subside quicker than thirst.

'The past few days had been very stressful and when I am stressed for a long time, I binge-eat, don't cook healthy food and eat all the unhealthy stuff I can think of. This time, though, when I went to the kitchen to binge-eat and opened a packet of unhealthy food, I asked myself if it was worth all the effort I had been putting into eating clean. NO, it was not. So I made a decision that I would not feed my body crap because I was stressed out. This time I told myself that I could not change the situation around me, but I could change myself. So I dry-fasted for eighteen hours and, instead of giving my body slow poison, I gave it rest. At the end of the day, I was happy that I was able to control myself and was at peace with the situation. If I can do it, so can you!'

—Kritika

3. It helps adapt to stress

Fasting is a kind of stress to the brain, because there is an interruption in the supply of glucose to it for some time. The brain then adapts to this stress by activating response pathways that help it cope with the stress and resist disease. Below are a few changes that the brain and the body go through during dry fasting:

- Nerves are protected during fasts.
- Nerve cell circuits are more active.

- DNA is repaired.
- The number of mitochondria to the nerve cells increases (exercising also increases the mitochondria to the muscle cells).
- More new nerve cells are produced from stem cells (at least in the hippocampus).

Fasting does good things to the brain, and this is evident from all the mappings of the neurochemical changes that happen in the brain. Fasting can also stimulate the production of new nerve cells from stem cells in the hippocampus. Fasting kills parasites and bad gut bacteria that typically feed on sugar, and this helps alleviate depression and anxiety.

4. Helps check brain disorders

Dry fasting is also extremely helpful in cases of epilepsy, because it kick-starts protective measures in the brain that help tone down overexcited signals that epileptic brains usually exhibit. Most epileptic patients experience seizures, and ketones suppress seizures. Fasting also increases the number of mitochondria in nerve cells, since that's the way neurons adapt to the stress of fasting. By increasing the number of mitochondria in the neurons, the chances of more neurons forming and maintaining the connections between each other also increases, thereby improving learning and memory ability. Hence dry fasting is known to be of great help in the case of Alzheimer's, Parkinson's, ADHD and other brain conditions.

5. Improves overall mental health

Fasting promotes not only physical health but also mental and emotional health. Most people report improved self-esteem, mood and vigilance, and reduced symptoms of anxiety and depression with a disciplined fasting regime. This can mostly be attributed to changes in neurotransmitters and the synthesis of neurotrophic factors.

Fasting also improves sleep quality to a large extent, which can also affect mood the next day.

Thus, fasting serves as a natural and free mental-health enhancer.

Spiritual benefits

1. Enhances the connection between our physical and spiritual selves

The practice of fasting is usually associated with religions reasons, but it affects us spiritually too. When we fast, it's easier for us to connect our physical bodies to our spiritual self. Without the toxins we usually put into our bodies, we not only give our bodies some much-needed break from the digestive process but also allow our spirits to be detoxed. After all, what feeds us feeds our soul too. It's common during fasting to gain a deep spiritual insight and experience long hours of meditation without feeling restless. Prayers become deeper and more enhanced. We become more grounded and humbled. Since during a fast we are not so consumed by thoughts of what we are going to eat next, we have more energy to devote to spirituality. Dry fasting also cleanses our chakras and gives a boost to creativity, with the resultant heightened awareness and brain activity.

Mahatma Gandhi himself practised fasting as a form of self-discipline and religious devotion. In Gandhi's peaceful form of protest, fasting was the most potent 'weapon'.*

No amount of surgery and medicines can heal a disease if the body isn't physically, emotionally or spiritually aligned; the body itself must have the capacity to restore balance. Dry fasting is one of the most powerful tools to attain that balance. Even a one-day fast brings about subtle and sometimes not-so-subtle changes to the overall psyche.

> *'After a dry fast I always feel something calm within. I feel a sense of well-being, a sense of control, a sense of rhythm, and a sense of synchronicity.'*
>
> —Sona Moorjani

2. Induces gratefulness

Most people who fast report that they can really taste the fruit when they break their fast. It's the same fruit they

---

* Whitney Sanford, 'What Gandhi can teach today's protesters', Theconversation.com, 2 October 2017, https://theconversation.com/what-gandhi-can-teach-todays-protesters-83404 (accessed 17 February 2020).

may have been eating every day, but being off food fills us with gratitude for the food that we eat and truly makes us appreciate it more.

'I feel so proud of myself after a dry fast! I never imagined that I could do it! But the positive feedback from people who practise it motivated me. I feel good; I have not lost any weight, but I feel great about myself! That's a real positive outcome for me. I look forward to a day of dry fast each week.'

—Swati Rai

3. Increases self-control

Dry fasting increases self-control too. When we fast, we learn to say no to the body's most basic and powerful desire—food. Simply put, if you can gain control over your body's basic desire for food, you can learn to control your body's desire for anything.

When we fast, our basest character traits are brought to the fore during the difficult parts of the fasting period. Lust, anger, irritability, jealousy and fear are just some of the things that can surface. But treat these revelations as good and healthy, because then you are forced to deal with them directly.

People often say that fasting makes them irritable. That isn't true. Fasting doesn't make you irritable. You ARE irritable. If you can learn not to be irritable while on a fast, imagine how much easier it will be on a full stomach! If you can avoid feeling jealous of others eating during a fast, imagine how much easier it will be on a full stomach!

8

DRY FASTING
AND THE VAGUS NERVE

One of the most overlooked aspects of the human body is the health of its nerves. Much of what we feel, think, talk about and digest, or even how two cells communicate in our body, depends on our nervous system. Hence, it is also important to look at our neurological health.

Our body has built-in mechanisms for maintaining good health. One such mechanism is the stimulation of the vagus nerve, also called the Buddha nerve. Each of us has twelve pairs of cranial nerves that emanate from the brain. The tenth, the vagus nerve, is one of the longest parasympathetic (state of 'rest and digest') nerves, which travels from the brain stem and splits into numerous branches linking the oesophagus, the voice box, the ears, the lungs, the heart, the kidneys and the abdomen, thereby connecting the brain and the body as one unit and facilitating a number of functions related to stress, inflammation, fibromyalgia, depression, anxiety, addiction to stimulants, weight gain, tinnitus, autism, cancer, multiple sclerosis and many other such conditions.

This nerve is thus connected to every part of the body and performs command-and-control involuntary functions. Here's what it does as it passes through every organ:

1. Originating from the brain, its function is related to depression and anxiety. Increased stimulation of the vagus nerve activates the parasympathetic nervous system, which promotes resting and relaxation.

2. On reaching the heart, the vagus nerve plays an important role in controlling heartbeat and blood pressure.

3. It then reaches the stomach and manages the digestive tract, contracting the stomach and intestinal muscles to help digest food and send information about what is being digested and the nutrients in it. It is also responsible for regulating the secretion of stomach acids, which is important for killing toxins, germs, bacteria and other pathogens that we may ingest through food and water. The right amount of stomach acid also helps in the digestion of proteins and prevents issues such as bloating, indigestion and flatulence. GERD, or gastroesophageal reflux disease, is also partly related to the vagus nerve, as that controls the amount of stomach acid in the system and the closure of oesophageal sphincters.

4. Upon reaching the gut, the vagus nerve plays a role in the secretion of digestive enzymes and keeps the digestion process smooth. We can continue to drink

jeera and other spice concoctions (which are great) but sometimes all we need is stimulation of the vagus nerve for better digestive health. The good gut microbes and serotonin produced in the gut play an important role in the stimulation of the vagus nerve, thereby sending impulses all the way to the brain. This is why patients suffering from depression and anxiety need to focus on fixing their gut health first. This nerve is also responsible for stimulating the intrinsic factor, a glycoprotein that aids the absorption of vitamin B12.

5. When the nerve gets to the liver and the pancreas, it plays a role in the monitoring and balance of blood glucose. Passing through the liver, it stimulates the release of bile from the gall bladder, which can rid the body of toxins and also break down fat.

6. Passing through the kidneys, it helps stimulate the filtration of toxins and regulate blood flow.

7. The vagus nerve has a critical role to play in the health of hormones too, right from testosterone and dihydrotestosterone (DHT) in males to progesterone and oestrogen in females.

8. Stimulation of the vagus nerve has also been known to be effective in cases of epilepsy, to the extent that there are clinics that offer electric stimulation of the vagus nerve. Small currents of electricity are passed to stimulate it and reduce the number of epileptic fits that people may suffer from.

It is thus extremely important to adopt practices that help improve the tone of the vagus nerve. The vagal tone is a term used to represent the activity and strength of the nerve.

While there are various methods of doing that, one of the quickest, most natural and inexpensive ways is dry fasting. It works in the following ways:

1. Dry fasting has an effect on heart function. It increases the heart rate variability (HRV), one of the key parameters to assess physical fitness and determine the body's readiness to perform. This, in turn, activates the parasympathetic nervous system and improves the vagal tone. Whenever the HRV is high, the vagal tone is also high.

2. The process of digestion is connected to the vagus nerve. When we fast, we give our digestive system a break. Thus, an empty stomach that has shut down its digestive processes signals to the brain to divert all energy for relaxation instead. This increases the vagal tone.

3. When we fast, signals related to hunger, satiety, blood sugar levels and any change in chemical and mechanical signals from the gut are transmitted to the brain via the hepatic vagus nerve (the vagus nerve that runs through the liver). These chemical messages help activate the vagus nerve. This, in turn, responds by lowering our metabolism.

4. Fasting also increases the levels of hunger-regulating hormones such as neuropeptide Y (NPY) and decreases the levels of satiety-regulating hormones such as cholecystokinin (CCK). This also stimulates the vagus nerve.

Apart from dry fasting, other ways to stimulate the vagus nerve are cold showers, chanting, singing, humming, gargling, yoga, deep meditation, diaphragmatic breathing, gagging, the singing bowls used in meditation, healthy socializing, praying, exercise and the intake of omega 3, zinc and probiotics. Since it is called the vagal 'tone', anything to do with frequency, vibration or sound is also a great way to bring about stimulation, activation, harmony and balance of the vagus nerve!

9

HOW TO SAFELY AND SMARTLY INTEGRATE FASTING INTO YOUR LIVES

Every lifestyle change that we incorporate starts with the right mindset—and the same holds true for dry fasting. Do not consider dry fasting—or even intermittent fasting, for that matter—as a 'diet'. It's a lifestyle. It is something you are adopting to change the way you live. You eat at a particular time, fast at a particular time and this has an impact on health and our capacity to prevent diseases. This is only possible when one fasts in a healthy and sensible way.

But when we make it a fad and call it a diet, it can do more harm than good. Fad by definition means something that becomes too popular too quickly, and something people start blindly following based on what others say. The moment we create a 'diet' mindset, we start to think of it as deprivation and starvation, followed by fear and unhappiness. This takes away all the benefits of fasting.

As we receive more and more testimonials, one thing I know for sure is that fasting can change human health. There is enough science today proving the impact of fasting on almost every disease biomarker. We have data from people suffering from asthma and how dry fasting has improved their breathing capacity by reducing inflammation.

The main research that comes across is the ability of fasting to reduce oxidative stress. Oxidative stress equals inflammation, and every disease today is medically thought to be due to inflammation—right from diabetes types 1 and 2, cardiovascular disease, cancer, Alzheimer's, dementia and Parkinson's to high blood pressure, hardening of arteries and kidney diseases. These are caused by uncontrolled inflammation in the body. Fasting has been scientifically shown to reduce inflammation caused by oxidative stress.

When we understand this science, we start to fast more diligently and not as per what people around us are following—16:8 is the most common pattern. If you are hungry during the fourteenth hour but push yourself for two more hours, it doesn't make sense. The fasting duration that your body needs can change from day to day according to the amount of physical work you do, mental energy you expend, the quality of sleep you get at night, and so much more. Sometimes your body needs food and you must give it that.

So, when you set your body to a perfect rhythm and a cycle of fasting, it will no longer be a struggle for you. But this will only come with regular practice. The more you fast, the more tuned you are to the needs of your body and its processes. Some days your body will ask you to fast for only twelve hours, and some days it will be able to go longer without food. Listen to your body and not a nutritionist, the social media or your friend. No expert knows the magic number of fasting that will suit you.

When your body is done with its elimination phase and asks for nutrition, you should feed it. Otherwise, you will only end up creating a stressful situation in those trillions of cells that are demanding nutrition, thereby producing cortisol and adrenaline that can be harmful for you.

The idea of fasting is—it doesn't matter whether you are fasting for two–three days in a week or a month, as long as it suits you. There are so many who fast every day, and that's okay too, as long as they feel healthy, experience no nutritional deficiencies and do not feel psychologically deprived.

This doesn't mean people who fast once a week or a month are any lesser. We know people who observe one day of dry fast a month to rehaul their body, and clean, detoxify and reset all functions. This is great if it works for them, because their overall lifestyle must also be clean.

10

COMMON MISTAKES ONE CAN MAKE DURING DRY FASTING

Dry fasting done the wrong way can damage our health instead of benefiting us. Here are some common mistakes people make:

1. Binge-eating during non-fasting days

One of the biggest mistakes people make is to binge-eat on non-fasting days. Fasting is not a cover-up for bad eating habits. You should continue eating sensibly on non-fasting days as well. This doesn't mean giving up your favourite foods. No. You can still eat your favourite foods in a sensible way, but not overeat. This is when fasting becomes a complete and sustainable lifestyle change. Sustainability is a huge concern if one approaches fasting as a means to cover up their bad eating habits.

2. Having coffee but still calling it a fast

' . . . But I only had a cup of coffee.' Well, I am sorry, then it's not a fast.

There are innumerable fasting programmes floating around on the Internet that allows coffee, lemon water, infused water, green tea, ice teas, etc. during fasting. Please let your common sense prevail. When you fast, you cannot put something as acidic as coffee into your system. You will only be harming it by doing so. Coffee is a burden on your kidneys anyway, and here you are putting coffee into your system when the ultimate goal of fasting is to clean and detoxify.

If you are addicted to coffee and cannot give it up during fasting, then don't fast. It's as simple as that. But consuming coffee while fasting is NOT a fast. It's similar with fruit juices.

The term 'dry fasting' itself means complete abstinence from food and water, and entering a phase of elimination. Let's be true to ourselves to experience the real benefits of fasting. There can be no cheating or shortcut.

Fasting done the wrong way will harm your body, cells mind and everything else.

Please understand that the right way to practising intermittent fasting is to consume plain water (no lemon water or infusions) and that to dry fasting is to consume no food or water in any form. There are no exceptions to this.

3. Skipping medication when fasting

Fasting is NOT a replacement for medication. It's an approach that's beyond medicine—meaning it should be something that you do over and above your medicines. If fasting interferes with your medication timings, think of a cycle that works for you.

There are genuine cases where fasting is just not possible because of regular doses of medicine every couple of hours. In that case, choose the longest gap possible and fast, but please keep your health professional in the loop.

4. Overaiming and overdoing

You don't have to fast for eighteen–twenty hours just because the whole world is doing it. Start slow. Maybe you can only fast for eight hours to begin with. That's okay. Next time aim for ten hours, then twelve hours— and that's how you gradually train your body and mind. This is how you do not make it a fad. You listen to your body and do what it asks you to.

For people aiming for a seventy-two-hour fast, first ask yourself whether your body actually needs such long hours of extreme fasting. I understand extreme fasting for people who are near death, some cancer cases, for spiritual reasons, etc., but for someone who is looking for general good health, why do you need to push your body? Challenge yourself with things like being a better person in life and being kind—not fasting.

5. Dieting during the building phase

When you diet and restrict your calorie intake during the building phase, it is not fasting, it is starvation. When you deprive your body of nutrients it needs, your body enters a stress mode—your sugar levels will fluctuate and your body will get more acidic. Yes, you may lose 2–3 kg but you will also put all the lost weight back on, and that weight will be ugly and stubborn. Do not try to challenge science and your body's intelligence.

11

KNOW WHY YOU ARE FASTING

What is your intention behind fasting? Most people don't even know why they want to fast. They want to fast because their friends are doing it, the whole world is doing it and they have a fear of missing out. If you don't have to fast, you don't have to fast. Keep it simple. Don't just do what everyone else is doing if you are already living a healthy life. People who are sick and need healing may need fasting but if you are fine and your life is going okay, then you don't need extra measures.

12

PREPARE YOURSELF FOR THE FAST PHYSICALLY AND EMOTIONALLY

Preparation is key to success in life. Just like running a marathon requires a lot of preparation, physically and emotionally, dry fasting demands preparation too. One cannot wake up one fine day and decide to dry-fast.

Before even starting to prepare your body, make sure you prepare your mind. Once you are mentally ready, the body will automatically follow. Here are some of the prerequisites to fasting:

1. Going through a dry fast is challenging on the mind. More often than not, it's the mind that becomes a limiting factor. Therefore, it's important to have a calm body and mind. Trust the process and the body's intelligence to heal. Having the right kind of attitude will determine how effective the fast will be and the extent of the healing crisis (detox symptoms) one will experience. For instance, if one is unhappy,

fearful or too sceptical about the fast, it will surely reflect both during and after the fasting period. Similarly, if one has a physical injury or someone has just returned from a long journey, tired and drained, struggling with jet lag, it is definitely not the ideal time to fast.

2. Do not directly start dry fasting. Learn and understand the principles and science behind dry fasting first. Read up on the literature, do your own research and practise intermittent fasting for a couple of days before going on to dry fasting. This will help the body adapt to the change better. The reason we feel hungry at a specific time is that we are used to eating then. Therefore, slowly prepare the body for a dry fast by doing intermittent fasting. Apart from adapting to change, intermittent fasting also allows the body to detoxify the system, so by the time you turn to dry fasting, your body will be prepared and the healing crisis will be more tolerable.

3. Wean yourself off caffeine and sugar before going on a dry fast. Too much caffeine can dehydrate you and too much sugar can only lead to more sugar cravings, which can make dry fasting difficult.

4. Lower the portion size of your meal gradually. This is very important in case of dry fasting, which is done for a longer time. Any light-headedness, dizziness, grouchiness or irritability that one experiences during a dry fast all come from glucose or sugar withdrawal. So cut down your carbohydrate consumption well before starting a dry fast.

5. Eliminate meat and dairy well before you go on a dry fast. This will eliminate withdrawal symptoms during fasting.

6. Having raw foods for a couple of days before beginning a dry fast is also beneficial so that the body can start to detox before you start dry fasting.

7. You can also perform different cleanses or detoxes before going ahead with dry fasting, so that the healing crisis symptoms are less pronounced. Detoxification before attempting a dry fast is crucial.

8. If you plan to dry fast for a couple of hours during the day or the night, adjust your routine accordingly. Make sure you keep dry fasting for days on which there is comparatively less physical exertion or those that are less hectic. Have a look at your calendar and make sure you do not have any parties or get-togethers planned that day. At the same time, try keeping your fast day a busy one, because it's easier to go through it when your mind is occupied with other things.

9. Make sure your sleep cycle is not disturbed before the fasting period, as most detoxification takes place while sleeping.

10. It will be helpful if one avoids exposure to the sight and smell of food. In Mexico, where dry fasting is practised for therapeutic reasons, there are special fasting incubators installed, where there is no food to be seen at all—there's only nature and positive conversations to keep one occupied.

11. Prepare and source everything you'll need when you break the fast—for example, clean water, dates, fruits and home-cooked meals.

12. Determine the type and length of fasting you want to practise, and be realistic when doing so. If you are a beginner, you may want to fast for ten hours; if you are an intermediate then maybe sixteen–eighteen hours; and if you are an expert, then maybe twenty hours and beyond. However, there is no hard and fast rule to stick to the duration. If you aim for ten hours but feel you can go for longer, then listen to your body.

13. Be aware of all the symptoms of the healing crisis you may go through (discussed later). This is very important. Most people panic when they experience a headache or a fever, but that's very much part of the process.

14. Make an informed decision with your doctor if you have a medical issue or are on medication that needs to be taken at a particular hour.

15. For patients dealing with low blood pressure or low sugar level, it's important to fast under the observation of a family member or caretaker.

16. Sustain your fast. A lot of times people give up in the first couple of days because of discomfort, and they think that it won't get better. Unless you have a serious medical issue (which you'll need to talk to your doctor about), breaking your fast before it's time won't benefit your body at all. There are a few

things that you can do to make sure that you complete your fast:

- Set an objective for yourself: Before you start fasting, be clear about why you're fasting. Is it for health reasons? Is it for religious reasons? Are you trying to clear your system? Remind yourself of your objective during the hard moments of your fast.

- Make a commitment: Sometimes it helps to get a friend, a trusted family member or an online support group to hold you to your fasting commitment. It's harder to break a fast when someone is monitoring you.

- Log your fast: Maintain a fasting diary for yourself. As you're preparing for your fast, write down each day what you eat, how you feel and what your objective is. Do this during the fast, so that you see how your body changes and processes the change to keep you focused on why you're doing this.

Dry fasting in the twenty-first century is something everyone should consider, whether they are looking to heal or to prevent disease. It is startling that everything in today's world is so adulterated, no matter how hygienic the food or drink may look. Going through a cleansing fast is challenging to the mind, only because we are used to munching and snacking all the time. When we are no longer able to do that, we get irritable. Hence, preparing ourselves mentally and emotionally is the best thing we can do before a dry fast.

Sometimes you won't even notice you're fasting. However, there will be times when you'll be ravenous and possibly have difficulty focusing on anything but your hunger. Being aware of this right from the start puts you in a much better mental state to cope.

Sample sixteen-hour dry fast plan (based on the circadian rhythm)

Day 1

6.30–7 p.m.: (Last meal of the day) Millet rotis, dal and stir-fried vegetables
7.30–7.45 p.m.: **Building phase stops** 1 glass of water
7.30–11.30 a.m.: **Fasting/elimination phase starts** Dry fasting (no water or food)

Day 2

11.35–11.45 a.m.: **Building phase starts** Sip a glass of water, slowly swirling it inside your mouth first (time can be extended if you do not feel hungry)
11.45–11.50 a.m.: Eat one or two dates/one banana
12.30–12.45 p.m.: Khichdi/dal and rice (a simple home-cooked meal—something soft and easy to digest; do not have too much fibre)

1–1.15 p.m.: One glass of water (keep some gap between meals and water)

Carry on the rest of the day as usual.

Please note:
- One can extend or discontinue the fasting phase as per comfort level.
- In the building phase, make sure you eat well. Do not diet in the building phase, else you will cripple your metabolism. Do not starve; it is not the same as fasting.

13

THE SIMPLEST WAY
TO FAST FOR A BEGINNER

The simplest way to begin your journey of fasting is to first decide on a suitable day. Have an early dinner (say at 7 p.m.) and you can easily build up to ten–twelve hours of fasting. If it feels okay, continue to fast. Else, break it the right way with due respect to your body—it will tell you how much you need to fast.

Indian culture, unfortunately, is one that has normalized late dinners. It was never this way. Our ancestors still used to eat well, in tune with the circadian rhythm. But today we have reasons like traffic, work and businesses to run—but, you see, the human mind always looks for an excuse to justify its bad habits.

With a few days of discipline, you can get into the habit of an early dinner. Once you start having dinner by 6.30–7 p.m., and eat breakfast the next day by 8.30 a.m., you would already have built a fasting cycle in the simplest way possible.

Feel free to play around with the timing, but fasting shouldn't be difficult. It should be effortless because our bodies have been designed to do this. It is natural to our bodies. What's not natural is constantly eating.

For beginners, the first few days may be difficult, because they are so used to eating. They may experience hunger pangs, cravings and irritability, but all of this will slowly but surely start to settle once you get into the habit of fasting.

14

FASTING IS NOT A COMPETITION

Never ever force fasting into your routine just because someone else has attained twenty hours of fasting. Let the process unfold gradually. Start off with basic fasting—be consistent, notice how your body changes—and gradually level up. I know it's easy to want to do it all in one go because we live in a health-obsessed society, but be mindful. People who saw the most remarkable benefits never competed with anyone. They did what was right for them—they went with the flow and never followed a rigid pattern.

What we see in social media is competition to reach sixteen hours, eighteen hours, twenty hours, etc. But that way we are just taking away from the benefits of fasting. The 16:8 pattern has become the new buzzword in society and everyone's aiming for that blindly. Please do not do that. Fasting is not a competition.

If you fast once a week and it's working well for you, and your friend fasts every day and it's working well for her or him, it doesn't in any way mean that your friend is healthier than you. You have found your perfect fasting cycle and so has your friend.

So, I leave it to you to decide whether you want to fast once a week, twice a week, Saturday, Sunday, Monday, once a month, four times a month or one month a year. Do what feels right to you. The end goal is to feel good and not trapped, restricted or deprived.

15

INTEGRATED FASTING (DRY AND INTERMITTENT): GET THE BEST OF BOTH WORLDS!

Integrated fasting is practising both dry and intermittent fasting in a safe and disciplined way. Nothing changes, except that you smoothly transition from dry to intermittent fasting. This works for people who can practise dry fasting for a short period (since it's extreme) but are comfortable with longer periods of intermittent fasting. It also works for those who want to extend their fast but feel thirsty after a point.

Let's take this example: You begin your dry fast from 7 p.m. in the evening and continue until 7 a.m. the next day. Then, at 7 a.m. you transition to intermittent fasting, which means only sipping water until whenever it feels comfortable for you. You still reap a lot of benefits this way and can go on a fast for longer.

Many people have been following this and say they feel incredible. This works best if you have to step out early the next day but still want to continue fasting. You may experience thirst pangs or if the weather outside is hot and sultry, you may want to avoid dehydration. This is one of the most practical ways to fast.

Conversely, you can start with intermittent fasting and gradually shift to dry fasting to extend your fasting window.

The number of hours you dry-fast and intermittent-fast is up to you, but this is the basic pattern. As mentioned earlier, you don't have to follow a trend—just do what suits you.

16

DOS AND DON'TS OF DRY FASTING

We have come across a number of concerns and confusions around fasting and its dos and don'ts. Here's let's summarize all of it. Consider this as your guideline to practising any fast.

Dos:

1. Make sure you are well rested and mentally prepared for the dry fast.
2. Try to start and end any fast with water. In case of dry fasting, an hour after you finish your last meal, have some water and then mark the start of the dry fast.
3. Ensure that you keep your mind calm and your surroundings peaceful while fasting.
4. Keep all destructive thoughts at bay. Deep breathing helps to stay calm.

5. Expose yourself to the mild sun early in the morning to get adequate sunlight.

6. Bathing is essential to remove toxins (if you are observing a soft dry fast). One can even do dry brushing (simply brushing the body with a specialized stiff, dry brush) to stimulate the lymphatic system.

7. Ensure you take enough rest, as it's important to take the workload off the vital organs of the body.

8. You can walk or do yoga/meditation or any kind of activity that feels right to you. For a beginner, it may be tough to work out, but energy levels after regular dry fasting only get better.

9. Stay busy and occupied with work.

10. Offer prayers, feel gratitude and practise meditation. Fasting is the best time to nurture your spiritual self.

11. Be positive about your fast.

12. Ensure you are breathing in fresh air.

13. Get a complete cycle of sleep a day before dry fasting and after it as well.

14. Break the fast with water and fruits that are easily digestible.

15. Slowly incorporate light meals into your diet.

16. Start with small and frequent meals after the dry fast.

17. One can also go for a whole-body light massage, which will help increase blood flow.

18. Yoga, deep breathing, chanting and meditation are great activities to do while fasting. You can even spend time reading spiritual texts if you want to.

19. Don't ignore your body's signals when you fast. Pay attention to how you are feeling throughout and

don't hesitate to break the fast if you cannot go any further. You will always have another chance.

20. Be around nature and prefer to stay in cleaner environments while fasting. While dry fasting, the pores of the skin absorb water from contact with the environment. This is one of the reasons many dry fasting experts believe it is best to practise it outdoors or in the mountains, as opposed to in the cities. The cleaner environment is preferred as the skin absorbs water from the moisture in the air. Sleeping outside and near running water is thus ideal for longer dry fasting periods.

21. Recite positive affirmations. These are positive statements that you say to the body. Your body is continuously trying to heal you, and you can support it and achieve greater levels of healing by saying positive affirmations out loud to it (or just to yourself). Put out this list of affirmative thoughts in a specific area so that you see it several times a day and say the affirmation/prayers with passion every time you see them.

Here is a list of twenty such affirmations. You can also create your own positive affirmations.

1. I have put my body in the hands of Mother Nature.
2. I feel amazing! I am amazing!
3. Hour by hour, my body is cleaning and purifying itself.
4. Fasting makes me happier and healthier, and makes me more energetic.

5. Every minute I fast, I am flushing out dangerous toxins that can damage my body.
6. I am in complete control of my mind and body during fasting.
7. I am strong and capable of reaching my goal.
8. I deserve and accept vibrant health and wellness into my life right now.
9. I let go of all that I no longer need. My body is healing quickly and easily.
10. I have abundant energy and a strong immune system.
11. I am deeply supported in my cleansing process.
12. Everything is happening at the perfect time.
13. I give up eating as a means of making myself feel good.
14. I turn to the highest power for internal purification and rejuvenation of body and soul.
15. My body is brilliant and intelligent enough to heal me.
16. My body is a temple; I have full control over my body during this fast.
17. No false hunger pangs will stop me from fasting.
18. My body is becoming stronger and I am becoming more balanced.
19. I will carry my fast to a successful conclusion.
20. When I end my fast, I will only eat what gives me nourishment and clean fuel.

In case of light-headedness, take a nap with your legs in an elevated position, or practise deep breathing. In case of bouts of thirst, practise pranayamas such as Sheetali and Sheetkari. They will restore temperature balance and help control hunger and thirst. Avoid this if you complain of excessive mucus or live in cold regions.

Sheetali

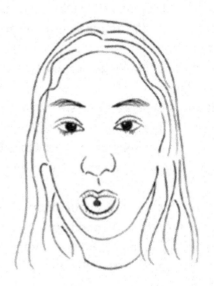

1. Sit in any comfortable meditation posture.
2. Close your eyes and relax your whole body.
3. Extend your tongue out of your mouth without any strain.
4. Roll the sides of the tongue up so that it forms a tube.
5. Practise a long, smooth and controlled inhalation through the rolled tongue.
6. At the end of the inhalation, draw your tongue in, close your mouth and exhale through your nose.
7. Listen to the sound of your breath as the air is drawn in. It should sound like a vacuum cleaner's.

8. A feeling of icy coldness will be experienced on the tongue, the roof of the mouth and the throat.
9. This is one round. Practise five–ten rounds of this.

Sheetkari

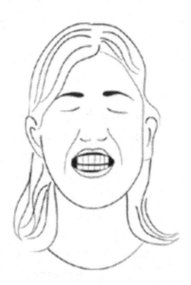

1. Sit in any comfortable meditation posture.
2. Close your eyes and relax your whole body.
3. Join the upper and lower rows of your teeth together and keep your lips parted (as shown in the picture).
4. Part the lips, exposing the teeth.
5. The tongue may be kept flat or folded against the roof of the mouth (khechari mudra).
6. Inhale slowly and deeply through the teeth.
7. At the end of the inhalation, close your mouth.
8. Exhale slowly through the nose in a controlled manner.
9. This is one round. Practise five–ten rounds of this.

Don'ts

1. Avoid drinking alcohol immediately before and after a dry fast.
2. Avoid stocking junk food at home, as you may give in to snacking on these when hungry. It's great to stock healthy foods at home.
3. Do not drink water, not even coconut or lemon water.
4. Do not take tea or coffee before or after dry fasting, as it can lead to extreme acidity.
5. Avoid smoking, aerated drinks or chips after fasting, as it can be detrimental to health.
6. Do not lie down all the time while fasting, unless you have any condition that might require you to do so. At the same time, avoid high-intensity cardio. Make sure exercises are not strenuous and reserve energy for day-to-day activities.
7. Don't take dry fasting as starvation; listen to the cues your body gives you. It's important to stop if you feel you are pushing yourself too hard or too far.
8. Free yourself from anger, fear and worry.
9. Avoid feasting after fasting. Heavy meals after a fast will be difficult for the digestive system to process.
10. In case of a healing crisis, avoid taking medication. Instead, lie down and focus on your breathing. The more oxygen you take in, the easier it will be for you to complete the fasting period.
11. Avoid sugary and oily foods after fasting. At the same time, do not 'diet' during the building phase.

One needs to rebuild all nutritional reserves with clean and nourishing foods.

12. It's also recommended that you cut off meat and dairy from your meals both pre- and post-fasting.

13. Avoid dry fasting while pregnant or lactating.

14. Children younger than thirteen years of age and people older than eighty should avoid dry fasting. However, short dry fasts for, say, eight–ten hours are safe. Children are more aware of the cues their bodies give them and will never eat if not hungry, so there is no need for them to dry-fast.

15. Avoid getting into arguments or quarrels. We will only demean the purpose of fasting if we do. Besides a physical fast, you must also observe a mental fast.

If you plan to dry-fast often and for longer periods, ensure you keep a week's gap between them. If dry fasting is done for longer hours, the body will adapt to it and be comfortable with it. Dry fasting will then end up losing its purpose altogether. Even religion does not support dry fasting for a long duration of time, say seventy-two hours, especially at the cost of your health.

17

SYMPTOMS ONE CAN FACE DURING DRY FASTING, AND WAYS TO HANDLE THEM

Sometimes things get worse before they get better! Just as a pimple needs to grow to its maximum capacity before it starts to heal, dry fasting can give rise to uncomfortable symptoms before it starts to show its true magic. Do not give up. The very fact that you are experiencing symptoms means that the fast is working. So hang in there!

These symptoms are collectively called the healing crisis. It is the temporary worsening of symptoms when the body goes through the process of healing itself. Fasting stirs up toxins on a cellular and spiritual level, and that brings all the toxins to the surface, resulting in days of discomfort. It's not necessary for everyone who dry-fasts to experience it. Some can experience many symptoms, some none at all. The intensity of the healing crisis depends on the level of toxicity in the body.

Here are a few common physical symptoms/reactions to fasting:

1. **Hunger pangs:** This is normal and mostly because of habit, since we are used to eating at a particular time. When you wake up in the morning, continue to do normal things. If you are soft dry-fasting, you can do oil pulling and brush your teeth, although it's recommended to skip brushing because the micro-receptors in the mouth may get activated and force the stomach to produce stomach acid—you want to avoid this. For most, things will usually get difficult at breakfast time because the 'need' to eat comes out of habit. Let it pass, just practise deep breathing and keep yourself busy.
   Cure:
   • Sheetali and Sheetkari pranayama will help with this.
   • Avoid being in an environment where you can smell or see food, and keep yourself busy.

2. **Back pain:** This may be due to toxins in the large intestine. Blood vessels that draw nutrients from the colon are very close to the nerves of the spine. Back pain will often decrease after elimination of the toxins.

Cure:

- If the pain is severe, apply warm sesame oil to the area and massage gently, after which you can put a heating pad against it to reduce the pain and soothe the back.
- Soak a flannel cloth (any cotton cloth) in warm castor oil and place it on the back. Cover the flannel with a sheet of plastic. Then place a hot-water bottle or a heating pad over the plastic to heat it. Cover everything with a towel and relax.
- Try and take an Epsom-salt bath to relax and reduce the pain.

3. **Bad breath, canker sores:** Waste passes through the lungs, which are organs of elimination. Bad breath will be a concern in every stage of a fast. Slightly offensive breath is natural and part of the detox process. Toxic build-up in the mouth and the absence of the washing action of chewing food can cause an increase in bacteria between the teeth. The tongue gets a whitish coating too.

   Cure:

   - Oil pulling helps overcome bad-breath issues, plus it also reduces the bacterial load from the mouth. (Practise if you are soft-fasting.)
   - After the fast, you can even chew on a teaspoon of fennel–ajwain (bishop's weed) mixture to keep bad breath at bay and digestion in check.

4. **Cold and fever:** Mucus is the perfect food for any kind of virus. Toxins weaken the immune system. When large quantities of toxins and mucus are in the blood due to a fast, they can cause colds and may even cause you to run a temperature.

   Cure:
   - Regular steaming helps remove mucus from the body. Add two–three drops of eucalyptus oil to the water and do a steam inhalation for five–ten minutes twice a day (with a minimum gap of twelve hours).
   - Application of castor-oil packs on the chest also helps loosen up the mucus, which can then be thrown out of the body more easily.

5. **Blackouts:** While fasting, the body goes into energy-conservation mode. The heart pumps slower and blood pressure lowers. Standing or moving quickly from any resting position will cause the blood to flow to the legs, causing blackouts and dizziness.

   Cure:
   - You should anyway ensure your posture is correct while standing or sitting, but during a fast it becomes all the more important. Move slowly and avoid jerky movements.
   - In most cases, this condition is caused due to lack of oxygen supply to the brain, so deep breathing would be best.
   - Lie down on a flat surface facing up. Raise your legs a little higher than your head; you can use

a pillow. This will ensure oxygen supply to the brain and you will prevent blackouts that can lead to fainting.

- If it becomes unbearable, then it's better to break the fast with lemon water with a pinch of rock salt to provide the body with electrolytes and improve energy levels.

6. **Headaches:** Toxins can cause muscle tightness in the neck and shoulders, resulting in tension headaches.

   Cure:
   - A few simple exercises to stretch your head and neck muscles can help reduce the intensity of the headache. Move your head upwards and downwards, to the left and to the right; then bend you neck towards the shoulders from side to side. You can also try to slowly rotate the neck in clockwise and anticlockwise directions to help the shoulder and neck muscles relax.
   - Eucalyptus-oil steam inhalation helps reduce headaches as well.
   - Take two–three drops of lavender/eucalyptus/peppermint oil and massage gently on the temples. Also, practise deep breathing to reduce headaches and make the detoxification process easy to tackle.
   - Applying an ice pack to the back of your neck can also provide relief from a headache, since the cold pack will help reduce the inflammation

that contributes to headaches. Plus, it will have a numbing effect on the pain. And believe it or not, just soaking your feet in hot water also helps get rid of headaches.

'I successfully completed three days of dry fast today. Fifteen years back, I would fast for three–four days a week. But then I stopped fasting completely and became a slave to food. For the past six–seven years I've had severe migraine issues. Every single day, I would get a headache in the evening. Skipping one meal was impossible. My lifestyle had gone for a toss because of these headaches. Managing two young kids was a challenge. When I tried intermittent fasting for the first time, I was not sure how I would survive on only water for sixteen hours. Surprisingly, not only did it become a lifestyle (I do it two–three times a week) but now dry fasting has also become a breeze. It's purely mind over matter.'

—Rajani

7. **Muscle tightness:** The muscles may become sore due to toxin irritation. The legs can be affected too, as toxins accumulate in the large muscles there.
   Cure:
   - An Epsom-salt bath provides magnesium directly to the body, which relaxes the muscles and reduces the tightness.

- Light stretching can help improve blood circulation and reduce tightness.

8. **Nausea:** When waste is released too quickly by the lymph glands, some of the toxic overload is taken by the liver and released with bile into the stomach. This causes nausea.
   Cure:
   - The most common tip we give our clients and one that has worked wonders is a teaspoon of ginger-lemon juice. This helps reduce nausea.
   - If you don't want to break the fast, then the scent of lemon essential oil or peppermint oil can help reduce nausea as well.
   - Stretching and deep breathing help in improving circulation, thus reducing nausea.

9. **Nervousness:** The elimination of toxins can irritate damaged nerves. Emotional breakdown is one of the symptoms that one can experience during detoxification.
   Cure:
   - Camomile tea helps in relaxation. (Have it once you break your fast.)
   - Omega-3 fatty acids may ease symptoms of anxiety disorder or nervousness and improve your mood by lowering levels of stress chemicals such as adrenaline and cortisol in the body.
   - Exercise will not only make you feel better about yourself but will flood your body with feel-good

hormones called endorphins. This always works in reducing nervousness or anxiety.

- Inhaling the aroma of lavender or tulsi oil works wonders when it comes to improving mood and calming nerves.
- A hot bath is always soothing, and raising the body temperature may help regulate mood and manage anxiety. For added benefits, stir in some Epsom salts. The magnesium sulphate in them has been shown to calm anxiety and lower high blood pressure.

10. **Skin irritation:** People with problem-free skin may have pimples or boils for a few days. A pallid complexion is also a sign of waste in the blood. When cleansed of mucus and toxins, the skin will be healthy, soft and unblemished.

Cure:
- Once the fast is over, keep yourself hydrated, try and drink three or more litres of water every day to enhance the elimination of toxins from the body.
- Apply grated potato or potato juice on the affected area to soothe it and reduce skin breakouts.
- Applying ice helps the pores of the skin contract, which prevents the accumulation of toxins in the pores that result in acne and pimples.
- Coconut oil always comes to the rescue. Apply it overnight to soothe the affected area.

11. **Tiredness:** Sleepiness is normal during fasting. There's no cure for this—just give in to the cues of your body. Try and rest as much as possible. Taking a hot-water bath will help you get a night of sound sleep.

12. **Low blood pressure:** Sometimes a person may experience low blood pressure during fasting—especially if they anyway suffer from low blood pressure. It is not dangerous.
    Cure:
    - A warm-water bath or a massage will make you feel better.
    - You can also do some light exercise to get some relief.

18

HOW TO BREAK A FAST

No matter how long you are fasting, the best way to break it is with nutritious, soft and easy-to-digest food. The fast should be broken with patience, calmness and gratefulness. Rushing into eating only does more harm than good, because the fast will have slowed down the digestive system. It needs to be fired up slowly, in the right way, to get the benefits of all the effort you've put in during fasting.

You could follow these steps when breaking a fast:

1. The first step is to thank your body for supporting you throughout the fast.
2. Then drink 150–200 ml of water sip by sip. Swirl it around in your mouth for a few seconds and then swallow.
3. Next, eat two–three dates and chew every bite well. If you are running out of dates, banana, figs or dried

apricots also work well. This will help line your stomach walls.

4. At this point, many do not feel so hungry, and that's fine. Respect your hunger because your body is still in detoxification mode.

5. After an hour or so, you may go for some fresh-cut fruits, along with nuts and seeds, buttermilk, lemon water, coconut water, kokum juice, jeera water, barley water or simply whole fruits. Avoid fruit juice.

6. Follows this up with home-cooked, simple and small meals such as khichdi, lentil and rice, soup or your traditional balanced diet after an hour or so. Avoid overeating.

7. When breaking a fast, begin with small frequent meals, gradually progressing towards larger meals with more time in between them until you reach a 'normal' eating routine, such as three meals a day and one or two snacks in a day's time. This is how one can resume normal eating patterns.

The right way to eat meals:

1. Eating slowly will help you chew food better, which leads to better digestion. The process of digestion starts in the mouth, as saliva contains digestive enzymes; so the longer we chew, the more time these enzymes get to act on the food, making digestion easier on the stomach. Chew until the food in your mouth is almost liquefied or has lost all its texture.

Finish chewing and swallowing completely before taking another bite. This is a good habit to inculcate.

2. Avoid tea or coffee at this point. Avoid glucose drinks too. Instead, have lemon water with jaggery or raw honey and a pinch of pink Himalayan salt.

3. Once comfortable in a day or two, add live enzymes and good bacteria to your system. Fresh, raw food is full of living enzymes good for the body and for digestion. Probiotics or 'good' bacteria are present in naturally cultured and fermented food products, such as curd, overnight soaked rice, buttermilk, sauerkraut, kimchi or simply fermented vegetables.

With practice, you will understand your system and what works best for you. Then you can use the method that suits you the most when breaking a fast.

19

DO NOT DIET WHILE FASTING

Many people tend to diet while fasting—they have skimpy meals during their building phase, thinking that this approach will help them lose weight faster.

Please understand this is wrong. In fact, this is harmful. The fact that your body has reached a point where it needs to break the fast means that every cell in your body is screaming for nutrition. All the cells act like a sponge—ready to accept nutrients. It's called the 'building phase' for a reason. Disrespecting that can lead to serious nutritional deficiencies.

Just like mindfulness is an important ingredient to knowing how and when to break a fast, it's also necessary to use mindfulness when it comes to knowing what to eat and how much during the building phase.

Do not overeat, but do not undereat or undernourish yourself either.

20

FREQUENCY AND DURATION OF A FAST

While some embrace it as a lifestyle (and this tends to be particularly true of those who restrict their eating to a specific window in the day, as in the case of those who follow Jainism), it's important to respect the science and principle behind dry fasting and not abuse it.

The frequency and duration of a dry fast—or any fast, for that matter—should be an individual call, because everybody is different and so are the functions of different kinds of fasts. It's crucial to be mindful about your own body and the signals it gives you to be able to know when to break the fast. A body that's toxic may need a longer detoxification phase than a body that's less toxic.

Some days you may need to fast for longer and some days not. Most people try to aim for a 16:8 fasting pattern because of the way the Internet portrays and talks about it. However, 16:8 is just a number, and no one but your body can decide its own perfect routine.

Use fasting as a smart and intelligent tool whenever you feel your body needs it. It could be after a weekend, or a holiday, or travel, or a wedding function or a birthday, or just as a means to recover from an illness.

How long a person should dry-fast depends on his nature and his body's needs. Therefore, there is no special rule regarding this.

The duration of a fast is never a hard and fast rule. One should start small and gradually increase the number of fasting hours, depending on one's lifestyle and comfort level.

Break a fast by listening to the body's cues, such as:

1. When you feel a slight pain or discomfort in the throat and the mouth. This is called physical hunger.
2. When the white coat that appears on the tongue during the fasting phase clears up.
3. When the taste of breath becomes sweet.
4. When the mouth no longer tastes as it did during fasting. It will feel cleaner and sweeter.
5. When the blood pressure and resting heart rate return to normal (BP: 120/80 mmHg; RHR: 60–100 bpm, depending on the person's physical condition and age).
6. When the skin becomes soft and supple.
7. When the body temperature comes back to normal.
8. When the body begins to feel light and internally energized.
9. When you start experiencing true physical hunger.

However, not everyone reaches this stage and could still want to break the fast much before they experience these signs. That's fine. With regular practice and gradual increase in the fasting period, you will experience this.

A word of caution: Be careful not to fast too frequently; allow your body sufficient time to rebuild its nutritional reserves.

'Knowing yourself is crucial to good health. I totally believe in this. I would like to share my experience of thirty-six long hours of dry fast. Luke, my main motivation were two things. First, after watching the many videos posted by you, my determination to take up a dry fast strengthened. Secondly, I was waiting for a special day to start my dry fast. I was preparing myself for it over the past one week by doing sixteen–twenty-two hours of intermittent fasting. As a devotee of Lord Shiva, I chose to start my dry fast on the auspicious day of Maha Shivratri. I could go without food and water for twenty-four hours without too many hunger pangs. During the day, my body would make feeble attempts at getting me to eat. However, after my twenty-four-hour fast, I didn't have to do anything to control my appetite—it vanished on its own. It was as if my body (ego) had finally accepted that I wasn't going to eat. At night, instead of winding down for the day,

my brain kicked into life. Ideas were flowing so freely I couldn't keep up with them. Not only that, I felt calm and serene. Before going to bed, I read a few passages from a book. Normally, when I read a book I have to use my intellect to process the information. But this time the words leapt out of the page. I didn't have to ponder their meaning or reread sentences. I almost didn't want to go to sleep because I felt so alive. I went to bed late in the night, feeling more relaxed than I had in many months, and slept so deeply. Today I woke up early and looked at myself in the mirror. I could see that long-lost glow in my face, and my mind was still so clear.'

—Anitha Pisharam

21

CONTRAINDICATIONS

If you fall into any of the following categories, it's best to avoid dry fasting or at least seek medical advice and do it under supervision:

1. Throughout pregnancy.
2. During breast-feeding, at least for the first six months. After that, make sure you are eating well during the building phase.
3. If you have abnormal levels of sodium or potassium in your body.
4. If you have high intraocular pressure. Please make an informed decision with your doctor in this case.
5. If you are on certain medicines that need to be taken at a particular time.
6. If you have thyroid issues. Avoid prolonged fasting, as it can turn on the 'fight or flight' mode of the body that decreases thyroxine secretion. Short dry fasts with the support of lifestyle changes are better.

7. If you are severely underweight.
8. If you have widely fluctuating sugar levels.
9. If you are suffering from kidney issues, especially kidney stones, UTI infections or are on restricted water intake.
10. If you have fertility issues and are trying to conceive (if you are practising a dry fast then, do so under supervision).
11. If you have chronic fatigue.
12. If you have been diagnosed with any eating disorder, such as bulimia and anorexia nervosa.
13. If you have chronic stress.

22

CIRCADIAN-RHYTHM FASTING: THE PERFECT FAST THAT'S CHANGING LIVES

The most common questions we receive regarding fasting, whether intermittent or dry, or both, are:

1. How many hours should I fast?
2. What is the prefect fasting window?
3. When should I start and break my fast?
4. Why am I not seeing results even after fasting regularly? Where am I going wrong?

While there are as many perfect fasts as there are people doing them, the one that's closest to the rhythm of nature is what I prefer.

What does that mean?

Each of us are products of nature and we thrive when we act according to its rhythm. The most basic daily rhythm we live by is the sleep-wakefulness cycle, or the circadian rhythm, which is related to the cycle of the sun. It's what makes us feel sleepy when the sun sets and awake when the sun rises. This also governs the way we live, eat, digest, secrete the right hormones at the right time, etc. This makes it extremely important for us to live as close to nature as possible. The more we move away from or challenge nature, the more we open the gates to bad health.

Now, fasting that is in complete alignment with our circadian rhythm is what seems to be the most beneficial for us. The habit of fasting is actually inbuilt in the animal kingdom, including us, and we have, for centuries, been following it—right until there became a 24x7 availability of food and electricity. In the past, humans would start their fast right after sunset, because there was no light or electricity to compensate for it, and neither any facility to store food. The fast, thus, spilt over to the next day until about sunrise, when early man would step out to hunt, followed by a period of feasting. This automatically led to a complete twelve-hour (or longer) cycle of fasting.

What does the perfect fast look like?

A simple twelve-hour fast in complete sync with our circadian rhythm is usually what I would call the perfect fast.

For that, align your dinner as close to sunset as possible—say, around 6.30–7 p.m. (or whenever the sun sets in your area)—and go on until the next day's sunrise (around 6.30–7 a.m.), giving your body a complete twelve-hour fasting period and allowing it to repair, recycle, rejuvenate, detox and reduce inflammation. This is a nature-induced pattern of fasting and not man-made, and is the perfect way to fast because it aligns us with the circadian rhythm or the clock of nature. You don't necessarily have to eat by sunrise—just listen to your body and feed it when it really asks for food. For most, a light snack like a fruit and a handful of nuts in the morning, followed by a full meal by lunch or noon works best. This is actually the best practice, because by noon your metabolic rate is at its peak, so your body can best digest larger meals. This also means that if one wishes to indulge in a dessert, afternoon is the best time for it.

Our circadian rhythm makes it clear why our bodies are able to do certain things better during certain times of the day. For instance, we perform better at sports in the afternoon; we sleep better in the evening, when our melatonin levels are higher; we have our highest blood pressure spike in the morning, which is why we see more heart attacks happening in the morning.

More and more scientific research is showing that twelve hours of fast that's in line with our circadian rhythm is more powerful than fourteen–eighteen hours of fast done at a different time every day.

It's very easy for us to abuse fasting and make it a fad. We party late and then decide to start intermittent fasting at 2 a.m. The next day we have another social event and, once again, this pattern is repeated. This way, even if we are fasting, we may not be gaining any benefits because it is in no way aligned to our circadian rhythm; plus the body needs more time to clean up all the alcohol and far-from-healthy food. Ideally, our body doesn't need so much time to clean up and detoxify. It can do everything

'I started intermittent fasting in September 2017, when I was 62–63 kg.

I lost 8 kg in eight months and reached a plateau, but could easily maintain that weight. Since I started the circadian intermittent fasting from May this year, I have quickly dropped another 4–5 kg. I started losing mad inches (still shrinking) in less than a week, with better and deeper sleep, less inflammation and puffiness. Now my weight fluctuates between 49–50 kg, and I feel great. I am now effortlessly maintaining my health and my weight doesn't fluctuate. I eat everything, including a dessert after lunch. I do this religiously and intermittent fasting has become a very easy lifestyle for me. I was in Mumbai from 17–26 October, but it didn't change anything—I could continue with my fasting as I normally do. Thank you, Luke, for being our guardian angel and for your love and concern for humanity.'

—Kavita Shroff

in a twelve-hour fasting frame. But the more toxins we add to our system, the longer we may have to fast.

How is this sunrise-to-sunset fasting beneficial for us?

Every human being has an inbuilt biological clock. The times we wake up, sleep, eat, digest food and secrete hormones work according to this clock. It's not a physical clock, like a watch, which dictates how our life should run according to external circumstances such as meetings, programmes, social calendars, etc. Our biological clock works according to natural markers, such as sunrise, sunset, the amount or intensity of sunlight and changes in weather. Our body functions based on these aspects and not according to what we decide as per our convenience.

A growing body of research suggests that our bodies at at their functional best when we align our eating patterns to our circadian rhythm—the innate twenty-four-hour cycle that tells our bodies when to wake up, when to eat and when to fall asleep. Chronic disruption of this rhythm—by eating late meals or nibbling on midnight snacks, for example—could be a recipe for weight gain and metabolic trouble. So it's not just about what we eat but when we eat that matters. At night, the lack of sunlight (darkness) is a signal for our brains to release melatonin, which prepares us for sleep. Eating late in the evening sends a contradictory signal to the clocks in the rest of our body saying it's still daytime—which, in turn, can not only disrupt sleep but also digestion.

Once we start respecting our biological clock and living in sync with it, half of the things human beings do today to foster good healthy, lose weight and look good will automatically be done by the body.

'I always thought I wouldn't be able to go beyond twelve hours of intermittent fasting. But over the last two weeks I have gradually challenged myself to increase the fasting hours by eating an early dinner. I took the first week to get used to my schedule but the week after I had dinner between 7 p.m. and 7.30 p.m. each day and breakfast between 11.30 a.m. and noon. As a result:

1. My energy levels have been amazing throughout the days.
2. I have not experienced any post-lunch sluggishness, and there has been a sense of calm that I felt, which I can't explain in words.
3. I was able to do yoga while being on a sixteen-hour intermittent fast.
4. I see that my skin has cleared up (I also do oil pulling every alternate day).
5. My weighing scale has been so kind to me! It came down by 1.5 kg.
6. Most importantly, I have been very happy!

Thank you, Luke Coutinho, for keeping us motivated.'

—Nupur Gupta

This way of fasting is also called the circadian-rhythm fasting, and is the right way to fast, because it's exactly how nature designed us to be. It should take away all the fads around fasting.

As a beginner, one must start aligning one's fasting cycle with this (around twelve hours of fasting) and gradually extend to thirteen, fourteen or fifteen hours and so on, until they start to experience true physical hunger. It's necessary to get fasting right at the grassroots level before one starts to aim for long and extended fasts. Most of us have the basics wrong.

This simple circadian-rhythm fasting is simple, doable and gets you all the results that you might be looking for in a fast.

We discovered this way of fasting (which has actually always existed) and the outcomes have been fantastic. People have reported:

1. Better sleep quality.
2. Complete relief from water retention and bloating.
3. Waking up with flatter tummies.
4. Not waking up feeling heavy.
5. Cases of irritable bowel syndrome and other digestion-related issues have got better.
6. Tolerance towards gluten has got better.

If you are a beginner, circadian-rhythm fasting is the best way to go. You can start off your journey with eating an early dinner, give a twelve-hour gap of fasting and within that drink just water, which basically means intermittent fasting, and then slowly step up to dry fasting. Or one could just keep it to intermittent fasting. Whatever works for an individual is what they should go for. The idea is to align your fasting cycle to the circadian rhythm.

So circadian-rhythm fasting in a nutshell is about eating your last meal (dinner) by sunset or as close to it as possible, then beginning your fasting period, which could be dry or intermittent, and then breaking your fast by sunrise or extending it if your body permits.

You can easily clock twelve hours if you follow this pattern of fasting—which is simple, natural, realistic, sustainable and, most importantly, effective.

FAQS

Q1. I am new to fasting. How do I begin?

Start small. Begin with short intermittent fasts, then short
dry fasts and gradually work your way up.

**Q2. I need to have my thyroid medication in the morning.
How can I approach dry fasting?**

Schedule your dry fasting accordingly, then. You could
begin it early, say post lunch, and break it in the morning
the next day with your medicine.

Q3. I am lactating. Can I dry-fast?

No, enjoy your lactation phase and feed your body well
with quality nutrients.

Q4. I am pregnant. Can I dry-fast?

Well, not ideally, but if you eat dinner well on time and breakfast the next morning, it's already a dry fast. So don't worry about observing a dry fast separately now.

Q5. I am diabetic and worried about my sugar levels hitting rock bottom if I dry-fast. Is it safe for me?

Yes, it's safe, unless your readings fluctuate a lot or you are insulin-dependent. You can start dry-fasting after your evening medicine and carry on until the next morning. However, everybody is different, so if at any time you feel uncomfortable, break the fast. Make an informed decision with your doctor. It will be helpful if you could monitor your sugar levels regularly during the fast.

Q6. I am suffering from UTI (urinary tract infection), and drinking water is important to flush out the toxins. How will dry fasting help me?

Well, staying off water and food for some time will create a very hostile environment for the harmful microorganisms in your body that are the cause of the infection. So hang in there. Observe the fast but make sure you hydrate well during the building phase. Also, make it a point to wash your genitals well after urinating.

Q7. I suffer from chronic acidity. Will eating and drinking nothing for long periods of time not aggravate acidity?

If you are acidic, fix that first. But also know that we mostly get acidic due to toxins, frequent eating and a bad lifestyle. You can always start small and give it a shot, though. Simultaneously, build habits in your lifestyle that help you cure acidity. Get more raw and alkaline foods into your eating plan, such as fresh fruits, cucumbers, carrots and lemons.

Q8. The first urine of the day after a dry fast is painful. Is the burning sensation normal?

Yes, very normal.

Q9. I cannot stay hungry for more than two hours. I need to eat all the time. How do I even begin with dry fasting?

Dry fasting will teach you discipline. You really do not need food every two hours if you are eating healthy and balanced meals. Prepare your mind and start taking small steps towards dry fasting. Slowly but surely you will realize you can live without such frequent eating.

Q10. How do I dry-fast in the summers?

Observe short dry fasts. It will be easier if you include the evening and early-morning window in the fasting phase.

Hydrate well during the building phase and live a healthy summer overall so that your body isn't overly toxic in the first place.

Q11. I have fever and my throat dries up frequently. Should I dry-fast?

Yes, you should. In fact, fasting during common cold and fever helps boost immunity and recovery is sooner too.

Q12. I have a hard time passing motion the next day of a dry fast. What do I do?

Well, in most cases, dry fasting improves bowel movement. However, if you feel constipated, it could mean you need to check your water and fibre intake during your building phase. If constipation persists, have a spoon of castor oil before sleeping to get some relief.

Q13. Can children dry-fast?

Dry fasting comes more naturally to kids. They are more connected with their bodies and can read their hunger cues better. Children will never accept food if they aren't hungry because their bodies are still in elimination mode. This is one of the main reasons most kids are so fussy when it comes to eating breakfast. So let them follow nature and avoid imposing dry fasting on them. However, any age group from the adolescent period upward can practise conscious dry fasting.

Q14. I am a cancer patient but I'm not responding to treatments any more. Doctors say there is nothing they can do for me. Will dry fasting help?

In the absence of food and water, a complete change in the body terrain is observed, which helps tap into the body's power and intelligence to heal itself. Dry fasting helps confuse cancer cells by generating extreme environments that only normal cells can quickly respond to.

There are a couple of things that happen in a body during a dry fast that may help a cancer patient:

1. The body's energy is conserved so it can heal.
2. The immune system is stimulated.
3. The body's sickest cells (cancer cells) are sacrificed for survival. Hence cancer cells are killed and this significantly improves the effectiveness of the treatment.
4. Any inflammation in the body is reduced.

However, it's extremely important to make an informed decision with the doctor before observing a dry fast at this time. If the patient has diabetes or blood pressure issues, then it's a good idea to observe these levels regularly.

Q15. Can I work out during dry fasting?

You can engage in light activities such as walking, yoga and stretching. If you regularly fast, you will notice yourself working out better because energy levels really increase.

Q16. I dry-fast for forty-eight hours. Is it healthy?

As long as you are comfortable, it's healthy. Your body will tell you when to stop.

Q17. Can someone with chronic kidney disorder dry-fast?

It varies from person to person, and depends on the severity of the condition.

Q18. Can I break my dry fast with lemon water or apple cider vinegar?

No, have plain water only.

Q19. I am already underweight. Can I dry-fast?

Avoid. Eat healthy and well-balanced meals to bring your body weight within the normal range.

Q20. On the one hand, it's believed that we must avoid long gaps between meals, and on the other it's believed that not eating for long hours is considered therapeutic. I am confused!

Both sayings are true. However, we should consider dry fasting as a therapeutic tool and use it whenever our body needs it. Otherwise, follow a lifestyle where you do not keep very long or very short gaps between meals, depending on your lifestyle.

Q21. I have been hearing that breakfast is the most important meal of the day but while dry fasting I am having to skip breakfast. Please tell me how to go about this.

The saying that breakfast is the most important meal of the day may not be true for all. Please do what suits your lifestyle. If your day demands you to have fuel well in the beginning, do it. If not, then you can avoid it and wait for true hunger to set in.

Q22. Can I dry-fast every day?

If you eat your dinner well on time (say by 7 p.m.) and eat breakfast the next day at (7–8 a.m.), and make sure you don't consume water in between, you are already dry-fasting for twelve–thirteen hours naturally. And the habit of early dinner has been practised for years. So do it as long as you are comfortable. Dry fasting doesn't mean it has to be for eighteen–twenty hours. It can be for ten hours as well.

Q23. I want to adopt dry fasting into my lifestyle but I also love my lemon water with honey, coconut oil and vegetable juices in the morning. Where can I include this

in my lifestyle if we are supposed to break the fast with plain water?

You can still have the lemon water and vegetable juice sometime after you break your fast.

Q24. Can I do oil pulling during dry fasting?

Yes, if you aren't doing dry fasting the hard way.

Q25. Can I dry-fast during my menstrual cycle?

Yes, as long as you are comfortable. Make sure you eat well during the building phase to avoid weakness.

Q26. When is the ideal time to start dry fasting?

Ideally, a fast is not begun in the morning but in the evening. The reason is simple—the maximum fasting time is bracketed by your sleep cycle. As you know, night-time is usually when the body restores itself and heals from diseases. By fasting like this, you allow the maximum opportunity for the body to perform tasks.

Q27. My work involves a lot of physical exertion. Can I still dry-fast?

When we fast, we are meant to spend less energy as well. If your work requires a lot of physical energy, then fasting may not always be for you. The healing benefits of fasting happen when the body is at rest and doing minimum work. So plan your fasts accordingly, not just for the sake of doing it. All of us want to continue with everything we do and also fast, but it doesn't work that way. We will do more harm than good. Fast when the body does not have to expend much energy. And, as always, listen to your body.

Q28. Can I dry-fast during summers?

If it's summer and you are not entirely in an air-conditioned environment, be careful of fasting with no water. You might risk severe dehydration and electrolyte loss. Try intermittent fasting instead. Choose to fast according to your day, where you live, your health problems, your environment and the work you do. Fast when you need to and also prepare yourself that way. You don't have to make dry fasting a way of life. Your body also needs nutrition. Choose the fast accordingly and respect it.

Q29. Will I lose weight by dry fasting?

Dry fasting is not a fad diet, and practicing it with the wrong intention is only going to harm you more. The intention of these fasts is not to lose weight but to enable the body to lose weight by allowing it to detoxify. When we detox, inflammation reduces and the balance of the digestive system is regained. There is no short cut to weight loss. In most cases, people struggle to lose weight because they overeat, they are lazy and don't move enough, they eat less and punish their bodies with exercise, and no sleep or recovery. Please do not use fasting as a way to lose weight because you will damage your health. Even if you do lose some weight, it's only going to come back as ugly fat because you haven't really changed your lifestyle. There are NO short cuts to weight loss. Get strong, don't overeat and practise self-control and discipline. That's more important.

Yes, there are some people who cannot lose weight due to medical issues but the rest, who are trying to find short cuts to losing weight, please assume responsibility for your actions, the way you live and its consequences.

ACKNOWLEDGEMENTS

Gratitude to the Green Sheikh for contributing to this book by sharing with us his wisdom and his fasting journeys.

Gratitude to Taarika, a dear friend who helped me put all this together.

Gratitude to Mugdha, our research head, for pulling out solid research and case studies done on fasting.

Gratitude to my family and colleagues for allowing me to put this together.

Gratitude to the thousands of people across the world and personal clients who practised these fasts and kept sharing their progress with me. This made me believe in the power of dry fasting and the body's intelligence even more.

Gratitude to my amazing family and Sangha, from where I draw energy and meaning.

I would like to express thanks and gratitude to Sheikha Noura Al Nuaimi and her family for inspiring me with wisdom from the holy books and their connection with health and fasting.

—Luke Coutinho

Gratitude to Allah.

—Sheikh Abdulaziz Bin Ali Bin Rashed Al Nuaimi

TESTIMONIALS

Some powerful fasting experiences shared by people after a three-day global dry fasting challenge

'Gratitude, Luke. Not even in my wildest dreams had I ever thought of dry fasting, but because of all your write-ups and discussions on it, I was able to fast for sixteen hours. Earlier, I was very scared of committing to dry fasting but, eventually, I did. Thank you for motivating people like me. Keeping my fingers crossed that I will do it for longer hours. Inspired and motivated by you all.'

—Ity Saxena

'Hello all. I want to share my success story of sixty-five hours of dry fasting. First of all, a huge thanks to my husband, Prasad, who introduced me to Luke Coutinho and the Sangha family! Being a super foodie, I never imagined I could stay without food and water, even for a *few hours! But friends, one thing is for sure, the body and the mind are way smarter than we think! They just need a chance. I have NEVER felt this light and energetic in my life, even after trying numerous shakes, diets, superfoods and what not! Here are some of my observations:*

1. *For the first time, I understood the difference between the voice of the mind (simple cravings) and the voice of the body (actual requirement). It gets super easy to distinguish between these two as I can hear my body talking.*
2. *The body will tell you when to break a fast. There's no point overthinking! I am saying this as I planned to continue to dry fast for more than eighty hours but my body asked for nourishment and I heard its voice!*
3. *Whether we think we can do this or not, either way we are right! We are born with unlimited will. Just do it and keep improving.*
4. *I am a big fan of affirmations, as they can have a massive impact on our deeds. The ones that I used during my dry fast were 'I am hugely grateful that all my organs are working efficiently' and 'I love my life'.*

Not to miss, I lost 2.5 kilos in the past three days! Feeling fabulous.

Again, my heartfelt thanks to Luke. You are doing a fantastic job for humanity.'

—Suchita Prasad

'Dry-fasted for twelve hours for the first time! And this when I thought I could not survive without water for more than an hour. Didn't think I could ever do this for this long, even though it's nothing compared to what many of you do! Just happy that I could do this.'

—Pooja

'I found such a wonderful way to dry-fast with my husband today. I didn't tell him we were dry fasting until the following morning (it was my second time and his first). I asked him to push by just one hour to complete twelve hours, since we hadn't had anything to eat or drink since 9 p.m. post dinner the previous night.

He said he felt thirsty, so I asked him to suck on his saliva. We then had to do some volunteer work and he forgot all about the fast. Before we knew, we had fasted happily for sixteen hours, that, too, while giving back to the community! He is ready for another round tomorrow! Yay!'

—Priyanka Muley

'For those suffering from the very irritating and sometimes painful GERD, a couple of minor changes in lifestyle can bring an end to what seems like a never-ending ordeal.

In 2012, I was diagnosed with an autoimmune condition called scleroderma. It's a systemic condition that primarily affects the blood capillaries and the functioning of many other organs in the body. For more information, please google because I primarily want to focus on acid reflux here. As a result of this syndrome, the two major problems that troubled me were inflammation and GERD, and I was put on medication for these. Ranitidine and Omeprazole were the two major drugs that I was told to have for my battle against acidity. And though I, religiously and with utmost faith in my doctors, took them regularly, I was not very comfortable with the practice. I started researching about it and realized that regular use of these medications had major side effects in the long run. I consulted my autoimmune specialist regarding the same but his advice was not very encouraging. So I decided to stop taking the medicines on my own. But it did not last long, because as soon as I stopped taking them even for a day or two, GERD would come back again in full force. I tried switching to homoeopathy, but with the same result! And that's when I realized that I had to go to the root cause of the condition. As my resolve to fight this disease became stronger, I came across Luke's video on acidity. What he explained in not just one but in almost all his videos made complete sense to me and so the simplest thing that I started controlling my intake of was water—more consumption of water at the right time and in the right manner, i.e., half an hour before meals and, of course, more during the day. Believe you me, I was off my morning dose in just about a week. But for a peaceful night of sleep, I still continued taking Ranitidine! In fact, I remember writing to Luke for the same and his prompt reply was even more encouraging. Determined to get off my evening dose as well, I brought about two more changes. I started eating more raw foods and being physically active more approximately an hour after eating my meals. You see, sometimes for chronic conditions, eating meals two hours before sleeping time doesn't suffice! One has to move about more to be able to digest it. And that's exactly what I started doing. Also, my raw meals are more towards the evening, as I am a true-blue Punjabi and I believe in the 'breakfast like a king, lunch like a prince and dinner like a pauper' theory! I am happy to announce that after almost two months, I am off my evening dose as well. And except for an odd day of eating out, GERD seems to be a thing of the past. It wouldn't have been possible, had it not been for Luke and his incredibly motivating videos. So a big thanks to you Luke and the entire Sangha family, where every experience that is shared keeps an individual on the right track. Also, I am gearing up for #globaldryfasting now as I have successfully practised a few times in the last couple of months and want to take it to the next level.'

—Neeru Sharad

'Hey, a big thanks to all you people in the Sangha and to Luke Coutinho for your lovely wishes, suggestions and blessings. Was able to fast for eighty-six hours with water, i.e., choviyari aatam taap (three days without water), and complete all Jain kriyas (including pooja) at Shankeshwar Tirth. It was a challenge to fast and exercise control over my mouth and body, but with the family's, the group's and God's blessings, not only did I fast but

also did it without water. And I did it with double the
energy. The schedule was hectic. We woke up at 3.30 a.m.
and slept at 10.30 p.m. and were active throughout the
day. Even then I did not experience any tiredness. I just
felt refreshed and blessed. Felt super happy that I could
do more than I had expected from myself. I pray for good
health and peace of mind for all of you . . . Once again,
thank you so much.'

—Chandrika Dhedhiya

'Did my first dry fast of twelve hours. Opened the fast
with my thyroid medicines, and hot water with lemon
and honey. Then had fruit after half an hour. It was
tough going, as I'm used to nibbling. And I felt thirsty,
as though I had just left the Sahara desert! I was feeling
fine physically. I was aiming for fifteen hours, but my
stomach started growling around breakfast. Thanks to
Luke's informative videos, I know it could be because
of an yeast infection. I will get my Candida cleanse
done soon. For most people, twelve hours of fasting
may be easy, but I'm not one who can fast easily. The
support of this Sangha and Luke's videos motivated me,
and I'm glad I am at least on the right path for this
lifestyle change.'

—Kaushambi Shah

'Today I completed fifteen hours of dry fasting, and I'm
feeling wonderful. Generally I get acidity if I skip meals
for too long, but, in fact, it's the opposite now. I think I

can pull it off for longer, but since it's my first I stopped at fifteen hours. That keeping your body devoid of food and water makes you irritable is a misconception. I have not felt such calmness in a long time. There is a sudden clarity of mind. This is a great feeling. Thank you, Luke. I feel content.'

—Archana Singh

'Thanks, Luke, for showing us the path to wellness. It's not just me, but I am encouraging my family, my two kids and my Momzee (who is here for recuperating after her cataract surgery last month). My son, who is very aware of his health and of Luke's magic, agreed in one go, and I didn't have to convince Mom much, as she is a master of fasting and does it very often (which I now appreciate and encourage her to do as well). I used to lecture her on how it was better to eat properly at her age. But she is thankful to Luke for making me do this. My son, too. He must be thankful that I don't run after him with food early in the morning, as I used to. My daughter, who I am very sure will get up late, will easily cover her fourteen-hour fast as well. My husband is travelling but I will ask him to join in at least for a day for whatever time he can. It is a boon that the maid is on leave this dry fast. We can focus on how to perform Saraswati Puja (ideally we do the puja on an empty stomach). So fasts yesterday, today and tomorrow . . . Yay!'

—Sonu Singh

'Things I learnt during and after my seventeen-hour dry fast:

1. *I have done fasts before but this time I heard and felt what my body said.*
2. *I was free from gas (caused by not eating or wrongful bingeing) and bloating (caused by overeating).*
3. *I slept like a baby for eight hours after many months.*
4. *In the morning, I realized that I didn't need a glass of water to empty my bowels.*
5. *My mind was hyperactive and I was in a great mood. God knows why.*
6. *I had my first sip of water and first bite of food later. It had never tasted so good. So little food gave so much satisfaction, and I did not crave more.*
7. *I actually had water at room temperature (it's a bit cold in this weather) without warming it, which I usually do, and I didn't suffer from the consequent throat ache.*
8. *I am ready for my next global dry fast! Thanks and love to all!'*

—Garima Agarwal

'Completed twenty-two hours of dry fast and broke it with 300 ml water and a few dates. Then I had fruits.

I didn't feel any weakness, neither did I have headaches or hunger pangs. I didn't even feel tempted while making dosas for my girls (I love dosas). I did all the household chores I had. In fact, even after breaking the fast I didn't feel like eating. Thanks, Luke Coutinho and the Sangha, for the motivation. I feel good. I never thought that I could stay without water for so long, but the body knows everything . . . Grateful to everyone for inspiring one another.'

—Smita Shibu

'Dry-fasted for twenty-one hours. I feel refreshed; moreover, I feel a sudden change in mindset. I'm more positive than before. I think dry fasting helps in checking mood swings and brings you out of any low phase you may be going through by fixing hormonal imbalances. Thanks, Luke Coutinho and the Sangha.'

—Disha Sachdeva

'Practised sixteen hours of dry fast and also went to my power yoga class after thirteen hours of fasting. Apart from the other asanas, I could complete fifty-one cycles of Surya Namaskar. Didn't know I was capable of doing it without food and water. Thank you for making me meet this new, energetic me.'

—Pooja Gandhi

'This is my sixth day of dry fasting. I feel fantastic that I can keep my mind so strong. I can also run 10 km without any dip in energy!'

—Gazel Agarwal

'I want to share how Luke and this group changed my lifestyle for the better. I was a foodie and ate so much junk every day. I knew this was unhealthy but couldn't control myself. Food was everything to me. I loved pizza, stuffed garlic bread, brownies and samosas. I'm very passionate about cooking and started a cooking channel. One day my sis-in-law told me to follow Luke's channel. I subscribed, and that changed my life. I realized how simple it was to stay healthy. I have realized the importance of health. Luke became a godfather to me. I decided to make healthy recipes as well, since many people don't know the simple things needed to make a lifestyle healthy. So I decided to inspire more people. My lifestyle has now fully changed. Now I live for healthy food. I wake up and have three glasses of lemon-jeera water. For lunch, I have fruits and seeds, Indian tea with rusk and, then, for dinner, I have dal chawal and salad. I am able to exercise. I have no cravings. I do two days of intermittent fasting and one day of dry fasting in a week. I eat cheat meals as well, but without any guilt . . . A special thanks to Luke. I always pray for him and hope that he inspires more people. I wish him more success.'

—Anonymous

'I'm a junk-food addict. I eat between meals! Since I started following Luke, I have changed my lifestyle. Never in my life did I think I could achieve a dry fast of fourteen hours, with no headaches and no thirst. I was perfectly fine and broke my fast with 250 ml of warm water, two dates, two walnuts and some watermelon!

After thirty minutes, I had my organic coconut milk with a bit of saffron (hot) and a slice of rye pumpkin seed bread with a little pure almond butter! I feel fantastic! My angel, Luke Coutinho, how can I thank you enough?'

—Sonia Gurnamal

'Thanks, Luke and the Sangha, for all the inspiration you've given me. I just broke my thirty-eight-hour dry fast and I feel energetic. I did all my house chores and walked 10,000 steps. Thanks. I feel so positive.'

—Siddhi Gupta

'I have broken my dry fast after forty-four hours. I'm full of energy. I run 10 km every day. Here I want to share my experience of dry fasting. I feel calm and relaxed. I have no hunger pangs, no thirst. It's the first time I have enjoyed the calmness in my body; I love it!'

—Poonam Singhal

'Awesome experience. Just completed seventeen hours of dry fast. Worked out for one and a half hours while fasting. I was really worried that I might not be able to without water, but it was not as difficult as I thought it would be. It is really mind over body. And, magically, the soreness in my throat vanished overnight without any medicine. I guess it's the self-healing mechanism of the body. All set for Day 3.'

—Rasika Dhingra

'Good morning, everyone! Day 3 of dry fasting is almost over. I like the way Luke Coutinho has taught us to worship the body and encouraged us to follow some rules for the betterment of it. It's not as difficult as we think. It's a mind thing. You start feeling that one can control the mind in a positive way. Follow this community religiously, knowing we can follow a few things, if not everything, whichever way we can. There is so much to learn from different people across the country. My husband isn't part of the group, but he also practised the fast these three days—though he does say he has hunger pangs today. The fast becomes more challenging once you cross the eighteen-hour window. Thank you so much, the Sangha and Luke, for motivating and inspiring us. Right now I definitely feel more energized, full of positivity, and absolutely wonderful and healthy. Thanks and gratitude to Luke for making us understand what we are worth. Three cheers to our community group! Have a great day, everyone!'

—Monia Malhotra

'Third day of dry fasting ended at 9.30 a.m., after fourteen and a half hours. Today I had a glass of water with three dates. After some time, I had some soaked nuts and seeds. Then, at 11 a.m., I had an orange and a banana. Will now have lunch at 2.30 p.m.

Everything went so well. I experienced no hunger pangs or thirst. My body felt lighter. I could do all my household chores without any difficulty. I have come to the conclusion that it's all in the mind. If you know *how to control your mind, everything will fall in place. I had a big phobia of thirst and had a small bottle in my purse wherever I went. Now I know I can survive without food and water for at least sixteen hours and more, if required. Thank you, Luke Coutinho and my Sangha family.'*

—Seema Roy

'Broke my dry fast of fifteen hours today. Had 200 ml of water and then some papaya and banana. Forty-five minutes later, I drank one big jug of lime water. My unwanted cravings have reduced drastically.'

—Anita Singh

'Successfully completed twenty hours of dry fast. I could have gone on for longer, I had no hunger pangs at all. Felt energetic and happy. Broke my fast with water, raisins and fruits. Feeling accomplished!'

—Daisy Lobo

'Successfully completed three days of dry fasting. Such a soothing experience. Happy to have achieved my goal. My conclusions:

1. *Four dates are good enough to break a fast with.*
2. *Having dinner at 6–6.30 p.m. has a good impact on the digestive system.*
3. *Dry fasting once every week helps you lose weight and also regulates your system.*

4. *A person can easily handle dry fasting while doing all of their work. One has to choose the timings accordingly.*
5. *It gives you a sense of pride when you are able to restrain your hunger pangs—the greatest addiction in life.'*

—Poonam Chaudhary

'Hi all. Today was my third day of dry fasting. These three days passed as if we were celebrating a festival with rituals. Although I was not well yesterday, for the first time I listened to my body and didn't eat anything after 4 p.m. The magic was that I felt really good until late in the night and had sound sleep. Will be breaking my eighteen-hour fast in some time. In these three days, I had a lot of craving for ice cream and sweets, but it was an overall victory. Thank you, Luke and everyone here, for motivating me. Everyone's posts are really motivating.'

—Pooja

'Hi friends, I completed my fifth day of eighteen-hour dry fasts in a row. Feeling good, energetic and calm both in mind and body. No anxiety at all. I always have severe fibromyalgia pain and feel very tired, but since I started dry fasting, I can feel that my pain has gone down by almost 60–70 per cent and that I am more alert and happy. My swelling and bloating have also gone done so much. Feeling very light and have no cravings for any food, not even junk food. Thanks to all of you for such good feedback on your experience of dry fasting and to Luke. I will incorporate dry and intermittent fasting in my everyday life every week.'

—Yashoda Bela

'What I learnt during the three-day global dry fast:

1. Everything is in the mind. My body is neither hungry, nor thirsty. I can survive without water and food for some time.
2. No matter where you are and what you are doing, simple practices such as dry and intermittent fasting can always be done.

Finally, and most importantly, I have found a new family in the Sangha that prays and wishes only for the best. Thank you for all the support and positive wishes.'

—Harini Machani

'Hey, here's my three-day global dry fasting challenge experience:

Day 1: Sixteen and a half hours
Day 2: Nineteen hours
Day 3: Sixteen and a half hours

During the fast: High energy levels, two pounds of weight loss (which I gained back), no thirst, no hunger pangs, *and mild headache on Day 1. Days 2–3 were pretty smooth. Didn't feel any difference in inflammation.*

The day after the fast: Super-high acidity with a lot of chest and arm pain. I guess gas was building up.

Second day after that: I usually have chronic inflammation, but for the past two days I was able to sleep better at night without feeling too much pain.

Third day after that: Inflammation was lesser, and my mobility better. My throat troubled me a lot. (Is it a sign that the body is getting rid of toxins?) When my inflammation didn't go down during dry fasting, I was disappointed. That was my main goal. But a sweet surprise was around the corner. I felt so much better after two days of dry fasting. I guess my body reacted late. Luke Coutinho, where were you all these years? I wish I had met you earlier. I could have probably reversed my disease. I am happy and thankful that dry fasting helped me manage my pain level. Am planning to do it once a week or more. My heartfelt gratitude to you.'

—Praneeta Kumad

'I practised dry fasting for thirty-six hours. Surprisingly, I was not hungry at all, but I was thirsty. I wanted to be energetic as I continued with my fast but my body felt weak the next day, so I broke my fast. While fasting, I noticed that my meditation was deeper than on the other days. It was like the organs of my body were thanking me for giving them a holiday the first time in my life—they work for us all day and night, and this was the first time they were free. I feel deep gratitude for my body organs.

While fasting, I did a one-hour meditation session in the morning and one hour in the evening. I've been feeling energetic all day. It is important to keep yourself busy, though. Thank you, Sangha, and thank you, Luke, for encouraging us. I am able to dry-fast and reap its benefits only because of Luke. I feel so much love and gratitude for him.'

—Rupa Jhunjhunwala

'Hi, Luke. Just thought of telling you how dry fasting has helped me. I had a very bad stomach and had to visit the loo six times in six hours. But then I decided to dry-fast and continued for eighteen hours, except for a few sips of water, as I didn't want to risk dehydration. I was absolutely fine the next day without taking any medication. You are a blessing to all of us. Thank you so much for guiding us free of charge, especially in this world of hawks, where we have to empty our wallets for even getting simple problems addressed. God bless.'

—Jyoti

'I successfully completed my dry fast today. I started at 3 p.m. yesterday but had to break it at 5.30 a.m. for my thyroid medication. Then, at 8 a.m., I had one date, two almonds, five red raisins, one Brazil nut, half a walnut (all soaked) and a cup of regular tea. Then, at 10 a.m., I had a banana, a boiled beetroot and a guava. I can't believe this. I am feeling so happy and energetic. My stomach also actually feels happy . . . LOL . . . I'll have

my lunch at 2.30 p.m.—wheat/millet roti, dal, rice, any vegetable and some curd or buttermilk. Then will again start dry fasting at around 3 p.m.'

—Deepali

'It's been years since I've struggled with weakness, fatigue and brain fog. I have tried many things but nothing's worked like dry fasting! The first day was a bit tough, but I'm super-energetic today! Looking forward to turning this into a permanent lifestyle change! Thank you, Luke, and everyone in the group, for the inspiration!'

—Rhidhima Khanna

'First day I dry-fasted for sixteen hours. I was coming back home from Mumbai, and had severe headache because of travel and exertion. On the second day, I dry-fasted for thirteen hours but I still had a headache. But I am fine now—will go on for sixteen hours. Thanks for your support. Even my stubborn husband has started dry fasting. He completed thirteen hours today. Otherwise, he eats only raw food until lunch, even when he travels. There is no craving for parathas and bread for breakfast now. He likes the way you explain things in your videos. Thank you! You are changing my husband's mind as well.'

—Dimpy Manmohan

'Did three days of dry fasting for twelve, thirteen and fourteen and a half hours. No bloating and uneasiness,

just a mild headache on the first day. I am feeling so light and have a sense of satisfaction and happiness that I could complete so many hours.'

—Prabha Vincent

'Luke, hello . . . Hope you are doing well. Dry fasting for three days was spectacular. I feel so amazing and so much lighter. I have more energy. I could lift weights better at the gym. My skin looks amazing. Thank you, Luke.'

—Neeru Surana

'Hi, Luke. I really want to thank you from the bottom of my heart. I can't tell you what a miracle the dry fast has been, not just for my skin but for my overall energy levels as well. Earlier, I used to run 6 km but with breaks. For the past two days, I've been running 6 km without stopping, and I don't feel any energy drop or the need to sip water at all. I feel on top of the world! My abs are beginning to show, and this makes me feel amazing. At forty-five years old, I feel younger than my son, who is twenty-two. Even he says I look younger than him! Thank you, Luke.'

—Anonymous

'My three-day dry fast was such an amazing experience. My energy levels are super high, and I feel so nice within. The last phase almost seemed like a cakewalk. Maybe I had much more control over my mind and thoughts.

I am looking forward to practising this more often and making it part of my everyday life. Thanks a million, Luke!'

—Shivani Gupta

'Hi Luke, I tried dry fasting for the last three days and I feel wonderful. I never thought I could break my habit of having milk tea in the morning. I used to be sleepy and have constant headaches. I stopped having it after following your intermittent fasting, and these days I feel an aversion to milk tea in the morning. Thanks a lot for this initiative. God bless.'

—Sreevani

'I feel so much better since I started dry fasting. My eyesight is better and my eyes don't feel heavy any more. My headache has also gone. God bless you.'

—Nattasha

'Dry fasting helped me get rid of my shoulder pain.'

—Neha Agarwal

'Successfully completed three days of dry fasting, for the first time ever! Thanks, Sangha and Luke, for the motivation and encouragement. I never thought this was possible, as I am so used to my morning coffee. I did not feel hungry after the dry fast, neither did I have any cravings. My fast on Day 1 was for fourteen

hours, on Day 2 for eighteen hours, and on Day 3 for twenty hours. I love this feeling. Never thought I could do this.'

—Hemalatha Shanmugam

'Day 1: Eighteen hours. Day 2: Twenty hours. Day 3: Twenty-two hours. I'm amazed at the way my body has adapted to this. I had never imagined I could pull off a dry fast along with work and exercise, but I'm completely fine. No hunger pangs or cravings for unhealthy food. I'm truly grateful for all the motivational posts and positive vibes around the Sangha.'

—Feltima Dias Mehta

'I completed twenty, sixteen and twenty hours of dry fast. It was a wonderful experience. Feeling energized and positive. Thank you, Luke Coutinho.'

—Vidhya Naidu

'The three-day fast was a wonderful experience, which gave me positivity and focus. Only couldn't understand why I was burping and gassy, even though I ate my food slowly. Thanks a tonne, Luke Coutinho, for inspiring us every day. God bless you all. I am proud to be part of the Sangha. Bravo to all of you who completed the three days fast or more. Gratitude to the Almighty for everything.'

—Shona Sweets

'Day 1: Fourteen hours
Day 2: Fifteen hours
Day 3: Seventeen hours

It's because of the support of the community that I could do this. I craved water on Day 1 as I am used to sipping water all the time. By the third day, though, it was perfect. A group of five people from my workplace have decided to do it once a week— every Tuesday. Three of them have changed their minds—'What rubbish are you doing not eating and having water for so long?' to 'We would like to give it a try too'. Maybe they saw me glowing and looking really happy.'

—Seema Wahi

'My best achievement? My daughter completed thirteen and a half hours of dry fasting without any problem. She will try to do more tomorrow. So happy. Thanks a tonne, Luke.'

—Ruchika Kumar

'Day 1: Twelve hours
Day 2: Seventeen and a half hours
Day 3: Twenty-four hours

This is my first fasting attempt! On Day 3, after twenty-one hours it was extremely difficult. Was craving water. But like most of you say, it's the group effort that made a huge difference and made me stronger. Yes, I definitely felt much, much lighter. Can't thank everyone enough for the encouragement, and kudos to each of you here who have successfully completed the fast. Thank you is a small word, Luke Coutinho, for all you do! Taarika Dave Arya: Thank you for leading this from the front.'

—Samara Vemuluri

'Successfully completed three days of dry fast. Did it for sixteen and a half hours on Day 1, seventeen and a half hours on Day 2 and seventeen hours on Day 3. Feeling so light and energetic. Was able to do my walk and workout too, along with household chores. Since I fasted without water, I wasn't sure about my bowel movement, but the body heals naturally and has amazing powers. I had no issue with my bowel movement at all. I had the best sleep in those three days of dry fasting. I usually have disturbed sleep. Lastly, seeing me practising dry fasting, my ten-year-old daughter was also keen to try it, and she couldn't dry fast but she did intermittent fasting for two days for fourteen hours each. I am so happy and thankful for all the motivation that we get from this group and from Luke. God bless everyone.'

—Riya Modi

'Completed twenty and a half hours of dry fast today. As I was busy with household chores, I didn't get the time to even look at the clock. By the time I finished work, it was 3 p.m. I took some rest, had a shower and thought I could still continue for some more time, so broke it at 4.30 p.m. with warm water and two dates. Later I had a glass of lemon water with virgin coconut

oil and fruits such as banana and apple with some soaked seeds. Continued raw until 6.30 p.m. and then had green juice and walnuts. Since I wanted to do the third day for twenty-four hours, I thought of having jowar roti with methi, dal and some rice. I'm really happy that my mind, body and will are working in unison, and I would love to continue for the rest of the week too with dry or intermittent fasting. Thanks to all my friends in the Sangha for inspiring one and all with their guidance and love for each other.'

—Aarti S. Anand

'Completed nineteen hours of dry fast and broke it with 300 ml of water, a few dates and a banana. I had some more water after thirty minutes, followed by grapes and berries. Snacked on dry fruits and nuts. Dinner was two chapatis with methi sabzi and chicken stir-fry at 7 p.m. Started third day of dry fast at 8 p.m. yesterday. So far so good. Feeling much, much lighter. Energy levels are high. The best part is that I lost 1.5 kg and was able to break the plateau, which was really annoying me! Grateful to my body for letting me do what I thought was impossible for me. Thanks, Luke Coutinho sir, for this mass dry fast, and everyone in this group for inspiring others with various tips and experiences.'

—Smita Shibu Nair

'I completed Day 1 and Day 2 of sixteen hours of dry fast. Did only twelve hours on Day 3 due to an event I already had planned for the day. I have been practising this for the past one month, so this hasn't been very difficult. In fact, I enjoy dry fasting now. It boosts my energy and immunity, causes cells to recover, makes the body feel light, and gives me so much positivity.'

—Megha Goyal

'I did my first fourteen-hour dry fast yesterday. I am a person who can't stay hungry for too long, as it gives me headaches, but I was absolutely okay after doing this. I was slightly thirsty but I controlled it. Feeling good! Thanks, Luke, for the motivation.'

—Dr Preeti

'This global exercise taught me self-control. Luke Coutinho, you just opened the doors of profound calmness and self-discipline! Regarding weight loss, I must say my weight hasn't changed! Whatever I may have lost must be the water weight, but something is clean within. Looking forward to more inner power to heal. Thank you, Luke!'

—Jalba Gohil

'I am so proud of myself and everybody here who has tried dry fasting! If not anything, it was a good exercise of self-discipline! There is a sense of achievement in it!'

—Deepti

'I dry-fasted for four days, and they were amazing. I felt light, my stress levels were low, my energy level was high and I had sound sleep. I did not have too many cravings, I did my proper workout and have been eating healthy. Thanks, Luke.'

—Clotilda Carlo

'I could do twelve, twelve and fourteen hours on three days of the global dry fast challenge, and still find it incredible that I could dry-fast for such long durations. Felt very motivated by your constant guidance and inspiring videos. I feel light, energetic and at peace.'

—Priya Vakil

'Dry fasting has become an integral part of my lifestyle modification plan for the last three months. I do it twice every week on Tuesdays and Saturdays for sixteen hours each. My wellness mentor, Luke, gave me inspiration to try the global dry fast for three days, from 21 January, 8 p.m. onwards. I had never tried dry fasting for three consecutive days. But I participated in this challenge and completed the three-day dry fast challenge successfully.

21 January (Day 1): Sixteen hours, from 8 p.m. to noon
22 January (Day 2): Sixteen hours from 8 p.m. to noon
23 January (Day 3): Seventeen hours from 8 p.m. to 1 p.m.

Dry fasting is important as it heals and repairs our body from within when we give the digestive system a break. Grateful to Luke Coutinho for this motivation to do community fasting together on a global scale. God bless everyone who participated in this challenge with health and happiness. It's easy!'

—Jayanand Wagh

'I have been fasting on and off, but had never followed dry fasting until I watched Luke Coutinho's video. Today is my third day of dry fasting for sixteen hours. I feel I have broken the mental barriers I had. I was sceptical but after reading everyone's posts, I was motivated to go ahead with it. I suffer from acidity and migraine attacks often, and I am proud to say that the past three days have been the best. I'm more energetic and feel great. A special thanks to Monica Soans for introducing me to this amazing group. God bless everyone. Thank you, Luke.'

—Anita Karani

'I just broke my twenty-nine-hour dry fast, and I can't even tell you how energetic I feel. This is the first time I could manage a dry fast for so long, and this is the first time I am feeling so full of energy. Thanks, Luke Coutinho, for introducing us to this wonderful technique called dry fasting.'

—Disha Sachdeva

'It was so easy this time to hold the karva chauth fast. I did dry fasting until noon and then went on a water fast. I will break it at moonrise. Thanks, Luke Coutinho, for helping me discover I had so much willpower.'

—Preeti

'I completed twenty hours of dry fast. I could have held it for longer but had to break the fast due to an anxious husband, who was so amazed to see me hopping around the house like an energized Duracell bunny! I also completed my morning exercise and walked 10 ,000 steps. This is how I broke my fast:

1. A glass of warm water with a date, a few soaked cashew nuts and pistas with cacao nibs.
2. A handful of strawberries and blueberries with a tablespoon of almonds, cashew nuts and Brazil nut butter.
3. After thirty minutes had a glass of unstrained vegetable juice.
4. After an hour I had an early dinner (7.30 p.m.) of poha made with vegetables and cauli-rice (an excellent low-carb and nutrient-dense substitute for rice).
5. Realized at 9 p.m. that I still wanted some food, so wrapped the day up with an egg sunny side up and a turmeric latte made in coconut milk.

Thank you for all your inspiration!'

—Richa Walia

'Broke my first day of the global dry fast challenge at sixteen hours, with lukewarm water, two dates, a handful of seeds, almonds, grapes and pomegranate. Will have lunch when I feel hungry. This is such an amazing feeling. Cheers to us and a big thank you to Luke Sir and my

Sangha for their constant support and love. Much love and gratitude.'

—Pallavi Bhoirekar

'Dry fasting is the best way to remove toxins from the body. The first day was difficult as I was hungry and even had a bit of a headache. But the next time was better and now it's like I wait to dry-fast. This change has come about only in a month! While dry fasting, my energy level is good. There are no headaches now, and I don't feel hungry either. Thanks so much for introducing me to dry fasting.'

—Jasbir Rao

'I have been dry fasting for a few weeks now, about twice a week. My left-knee pain has been a constant for almost the past five years now, after bearing the weight of triplets during my pregnancy. It's always there. I also have disturbed sleep due to the pain. I have tried a lot of things to overcome it. I had anti-inflammatory powder, seeds, raw and anti-inflammatory food, and supplements. All this helped my D3 levels go up from 3 to 52, but the pain just wouldn't go away. Then I started dry fasting twice a week. I still get headaches whenever I dry-fast but I don't give up because the relief from the pain is phenomenal. I urge everyone suffering from arthritis to please dry-fast at least twice or thrice a week. It works. It's a natural painkiller. I'm nowhere close to being fully healed, but I know I can do it with dry fasting.

Just thought of sharing this, as I know arthritis pain can be very debilitating. Thanks, Luke, for this powerful weapon you have introduced us to.'

—Aruna Anand

'Namaste, Luke, all the way from Dubai. I started my dry fasting trial a couple of days ago. Today is the third day and I feel fantastic! I am still fasting, and I must tell you the meditative experience during the fast has taken on a different dimension altogether. I feel balanced and also high-energy. Thanks for being instrumental in this experience. I am forty years old and on medication for various health conditions such as diabetes, hypertension and hypothyroidism, but nothing could stop me from giving it a shot and understanding my body better. Cheers to a reset. Let's make a healthy and happy world. Way to go, Luke and team!'

—Kavitha K. Nair

'I have dry-fasted multiple times in my life. Every year, when it was Shravan or Jain Chaumasa, I used to fast on particular days. In the end, I did three days of water fasting too. I have had multiple benefits from dry fasting. I just have no words to express my experience—I can only say that this was an experience greater than any other I have ever had. Prayers for the world. I was at peace every moment. There was not a single person who didn't compliment me on the glow I had on my face. It was all new, I was all new. On the

fifth day, when I passed very black motion, it was clear to me that 100 per cent toxins had been thrown out of my body. I could feel it daily in my urine too. The next best thing was that my skin started peeling off by itself in parts, and I got new, illuminated skin as if my face was lit by a bulb. I can't even describe my hair. My spiritual and emotional self was at its peak during this phase. I became more humble and positive, the best version of myself. I thought I could write about this. It took a few days for my body to adapt to normal food again. Now, every year, I fast for three days at least in a row and feel very good for my body. For one or two days, I am a little low on energy but this bounces back to normal after breaking the fast.'

—Shilpa Jain

'I am amazed by the way you help not only your clients but everyone around the world. I live in California and am able to follow you just because of your approachability via Facebook. I practise dry fasts with the help of the guidelines you provide in your videos. I also practise intermittent fasting regularly. I have almost fasted regularly and I see a lot of energy in me. I cannot even imagine that I have so much energy to do my chores after coming back from work. I am a rheumatoid arthritis patient with other complications such as thyroid and PCOD. I used to be in pain all the time in different parts of my body. I felt tired and lethargic, especially after work. I didn't even have the energy to *cook dinner. However, now, after dry fasting, I am able to come home, make dinner, tidy up the kitchen and, most importantly, sleep well (which was a huge problem for many years). Thank you is a simple word to convey my gratitude to you.'*

—Keerthy Puttagunta

REFERENCES

1. John F. Trepanowski and Richard J. Bloomer, 'The impact of religious fasting on human health', BMC Nutrition Journal, 22 November 2010, https://nutritionj.biomedcentral.com/articles/10.1186/1475-2891-9-57
2. 'Fasting', Wikipedia, https://en.wikipedia.org/wiki/Fasting
3. Alirezaei M., Kemball C.C., Flynn C.T., Wood M.R., Whitton J.L. and Kiosses W.B., 'Short-term fasting induces profound neuronal autophagy', NCBI, 14 August 2010, https://www.ncbi.nlm.nih.gov/pubmed/20534972
4. Changhan Lee, Lizzia Raffaghello, Sebastian Brandhorst, Fernando M. Safdie, Giovanna Bianchi, Alejandro Martin-Montalvo, Vito Pistoia, Min Wei1, Saewon Hwang, Annalisa Merlino, Laura Emionite, Rafael de Cabo and Valter D. Longo, 'Fasting Cycles Retard Growth of Tumors and Sensitize a

Range of Cancer Cell Types to Chemotherapy',
Science Translational Medicine, 7 March 2012,
https://stm.sciencemag.org/content/4/124/124ra27.
abstract?sid=243335d1-0e25-4036-892b-
9f7a6eb9744

5. https://www.cancer.net/blog/2016-10/fasting-
during-%20cancer-treatment-it-safe

6. 'Scientifically-designed fasting diet lowers
risks for major diseases', Science Daily, 16
February 2017, https://www.sciencedaily.com/
releases/2017/02/170216103923.htm

7. Chia-Wei Cheng, Valentina Villani, Roberta Buono,
Min Wei, Sanjeev Kumar, Omer H. Yilmaz, Pinchas
Cohen, Julie B. Sneddon, Laura Perin and Valter D.
Longo, 'Fasting-Mimicking Diet Promotes Ngn3-
Driven β-Cell Regeneration to Reverse Diabetes',
Cell, 23 February 2017, http://www.cell.com/cell/
fulltext/S0092-8674(17)30130-7

8. Guillaume Fond, Alexandra Macgregor, Marion
Leboyer and Andreas Michalsen, 'Fasting in mood
disorders: neurobiology and effectiveness. A review
of the literature', ScienceDirect, 30 October 2013,
https://www.sciencedirect.com/science/article/abs/pii/
S0165178112008153

9. Thomas N. Seyfried and Laura M. Shelton, 'Cancer
as a metabolic disease', Nutrition & Metabolism,
27 January 2010, https://nutritionandmetabolism.
biomedcentral.com/ articles/10.1186/1743-7075-7-7

10. David Gutierrez, 'Five-day "fasting" diet miraculously
slows aging, can prevent death from heart disease,

cancer and diabetes', Natural News, 15 July 2015, https://www.naturalnews.com/050409_longevity_ natural_health_five-day_fast.html

11. 'Spirituality to Science and Atheism', Ancient Healing Secrets, https://ancienthealingsecrets.wordpress.com/

12. Arjun Walia, 'Neuroscientist Shows What Fasting Does To Your Brain & Why Big Pharma Won't Study It', Collective Evolution, 11 December 2015, https://www.collective-evolution.com/2015/12/11/ neuroscientist-shows-what-fasting-does-to-your-brain-why-big-pharma-wont-study-it/

13. Fernando M. Safdie, Tanya Dorff, David Quinn, Luigi Fontana, Min Wei, Changhan Lee, Pinchas Cohen and Valter D. Longo, 'Fasting and cancer treatment in humans: A case series report', NCBI, 31 December 2009, https://www.ncbi.nlm.nih.gov/pmc/ articles/PMC2815756/

14. Julia Ries, 'This Is Your Body On Intermittent Fasting', HuffPost, 4 January 2020, https://www. huffingtonpost.in/entry/body-intermittent-fasting_l_ 5e0a3220c5b6b5a713b22dcb

15. 'Diabetic mice on fasting-mimicking diet repair insulin-producing pancreas cells', Eurekalert, 23 February 2017, https://www.eurekalert.org/pub_ releases/2017-02/cp-dmo021617.php

16. Suzanne Wu, 'Fasting triggers stem cell regeneration of damaged, old immune system', USC News, 5 June 2014, https://news.usc.edu/63669/fasting-triggers-stem-cell-regeneration-of-damaged-old-immune-system/

17. Mager DE, Wan R, Brown M, Cheng A, Wareski P, Abernethy DR and Mattson MP, 'Caloric restriction and intermittent fasting alter spectral measures of heart rate and blood pressure variability in rats', NCBI, 20 April 2006, https://www.ncbi.nlm.nih.gov/pubmed/16581971

18. Puya Yazdi, MD, reviewed by Ana Aleksic, MSc (Pharmacy), '19 Factors That May Stimulate Your Vagus Nerve Naturally', Self-Hacked, 6 January 2020, https://selfhacked.com/blog/32-ways-to-stimulate-your-vagus-nerve-and-all-you-need-to-know-about-it/#14_Fasting

19. Chan JL, Mietus JE, Raciti PM, Goldberger AL and Mantzoros CS, 'Short-term fasting-induced autonomic activation and changes in catecholamine levels are not mediated by changes in leptin levels in healthy humans', NCBI, January 2007, https://www.ncbi.nlm.nih.gov/pubmed/17201801

20. Székely M, 'The vagus nerve in thermoregulation and energy metabolism', NCBI, 20 December 2000, https://www.ncbi.nlm.nih.gov/pubmed/11189024

21. Mohammad Adawi, Abdulla Watad, Stav Brown, Khadija Aazza, Hicham Aazza, Mohamed Zouhir, Kassem Sharif, Khaled Ghanayem, Raymond Farah, Hussein Mahagna, Stefano Fiordoro, Samir Giuseppe Sukkar, Nicola Luigi Bragazzi and Naim Mahroum, 'Ramadan Fasting Exerts Immunomodulatory Effects: Insights from a Systematic Review', NCBI, 27 November 2017, https://www.ncbi.nlm.nih.gov/pmc/articles/PMC5712070/

22. Asma, 'Japanese cell biologist discovers "self-eating cell" and how fasting helps our body win Nobel Prize, Good Times, 3 May 2019, http://www.gtgoodtimes.com/2019/05/03/japanese-cell-biologist-discovers-self-eating-cell-and-how-fasting-helps-our-body-wins-nobel-prize/

23. Rich Haridy, 'Harvard study uncovers why fasting can lead to a longer and healthier life', New Atlas, 5 November 2017, https://newatlas.com/fasting-increase-lifespan-mitochondria-harvard/52058/

24. Anne Trafton, 'Fasting boosts stem cells' regenerative capacity', MIT News, 3 May 2018, http://news.mit.edu/2018/fasting-boosts-stem-cells-regenerative-capacity-0503

25. 'Dry Fasting: The Amazing Health Benefits Everyone Should Know About', Tonywideman.com, https://tonywideman.com/dry-fasting/

26. Ana Sandoiu, 'Fasting-induced anti-aging molecule keeps blood vessels young', Medical News Today, 11 September 2018, https://www.medicalnewstoday.com/articles/323039

27. Mohammad Adawi, Abdulla Watad, Stav Brown, Khadija Aazza, Hicham Aazza, Mohamed Zouhir, Kassem Sharif, Khaled Ghanayem, Raymond Farah, Hussein Mahagna, Stefano Fiordoro, Samir Giuseppe Sukkar, Nicola Luigi Bragazzi and Naim Mahroum, 'Ramadan Fasting Exerts Immunomodulatory Effects: Insights from a Systematic Review', Frontiers, 27 November 2017, https://www.frontiersin.org/articles/10.3389/fimmu.2017.01144/full

28. Fahrial Syam A, Suryani Sobur C, Abdullah M, Makmun D, 'Ramadan Fasting Decreases Body Fat but Not Protein Mass', NCBI, 2 January 2016, https://www.ncbi.nlm.nih.gov/pubmed/27279831

29. The Mount Sinai Hospital, 'Researchers discover that fasting reduces inflammation and improves chronic inflammatory diseases', Medical Xpress, 22 August 2019, https://medicalxpress.com/news/2019-08-fasting-inflammation-chronic-inflammatory-diseases.html

30. Unalacak M, Kara IH, Baltaci D, Erdem O and Bucaktepe PG, 'Effects of Ramadan fasting on biochemical and hematological parameters and cytokines in healthy and obese individuals', NCBI, 16 January 2011, https://www.ncbi.nlm.nih.gov/pubmed/21235381

31. Steven Salzberg, 'Can A 3-Day Fast Reset Your Immune System?', Forbes, 30 December 2014, https://www.forbes.com/sites/stevensalzberg/2014/12/30/can-a-3-day-fast-reset-your-immune-system/#103296963c93

32. Stephan P. Bauersfeld, Christian S. Kessler, Manfred Wischnewsky, Annette Jaensch, Nico Steckhan, Rainer Stange, Barbara Kunz, Barbara Brückner, Jalid Sehouli and Andreas Michalsen, 'The effects of short-term fasting on quality of life and tolerance to chemotherapy in patients with breast and ovarian cancer: a randomized cross-over pilot study', NCBI, 27 April 2018, https://www.ncbi.nlm.nih.gov/pmc/articles/PMC5921787/

33. Catherine R. Marinac, BA, Sandahl H. Nelson, MS, Caitlin I. Breen, BS, BA, et al, 'Prolonged Nightly Fasting and Breast Cancer Prognosis', JAMA Network, August 2016, https://jamanetwork.com/journals/jamaoncology/fullarticle/2506710

34. Ruth E. Patterson, PhD, Gail A. Laughlin, PhD, Dorothy D. Sears, PhD, Andrea Z. LaCroix, PhD, Catherine Marinac, BA, Linda C. Gallo, PhD, Sheri J. Hartman, PhD, Loki Natarajan, PhD, Carolyn M. Senger, MD, María Elena Martínez, PhD and Adriana Villaseñor, PhD, 'Intermittent Fasting And Human Metabolic Health', NCBI, 1 August 2016, https://www.ncbi.nlm.nih.gov/pmc/articles/PMC4516560/

35. Mohsen Nematy, Maryam Alinezhad-Namaghi, Masoud Mahdavi Rashed, Mostafa Mozhdehifard, Seyedeh Sania Sajjadi, Saeed Akhlaghi, Maryam Sabery, Seyed Amir R Mohajeri, Neda Shalaey, Mohsen Moohebati and Abdolreza Norouzy, 'Effects of Ramadan fasting on cardiovascular risk factors: a prospective observational study', NCBI, 10 September 2012, https://www.ncbi.nlm.nih.gov/pmc/articles/PMC3487759/

36. Geoff Hughes, 'Intermittent Dry Fasting | Beginner's Guide', Get LeanerToday, 22 May 2019, https://www.getleanertoday.com/intermittent-dry-fasting/

37. Horne BD, Muhlestein JB, May HT, Carlquist JF, Lappé DL, Bair TL, Anderson JL and Intermountain Heart Collaborative Study Group, 'Relation of routine, periodic fasting to risk of diabetes mellitus, and coronary artery disease in patients undergoing

coronary angiography', NCBI, 16 March 2016, https://www.ncbi.nlm.nih.gov/pubmed/22425331

38. Seka Palikuca, 'Intermittent fasting: Can we fast our way to better health?', The Do, 30 January 2019, https://thedo.osteopathic.org/2019/01/intermittent-fasting-can-we-fast-our-way-to-better-health/

39. Aliasghari F, Izadi A, Gargari BP and Ebrahimi S, 'The Effects of Ramadan Fasting on Body Composition, Blood Pressure, Glucose Metabolism, and Markers of Inflammation in NAFLD Patients: An Observational Trial', NCBI, 18 September 2017, https://www.ncbi.nlm.nih.gov/pubmed/28922096

40. Fernando HA, Zibellini J, Harris RA, Seimon RV and Sainsbury A, 'Effect of Ramadan Fasting on Weight and Body Composition in Healthy Non-Athlete Adults: A Systematic Review and Meta-Analysis', NCBI, 24 February 2019, https://www.ncbi.nlm.nih.gov/pubmed/30813495

41. Salahuddin M, Sayed Ashfak AH, Syed SR and Badaam, 'Effect of Ramadan Fasting on Body Weight, (BP) and Biochemical Parameters in Middle Aged Hypertensive Subjects: An Observational Trial', NCBI,15 March 2014, https://www.ncbi.nlm.nih.gov/pmc/articles/PMC4003623/

42. Suhard M. Bahijri, Ghada M. Ajabnoor, Anwar Borai, Jumana Y. Al-Aama and George P. Chrousos, 'Effect of Ramadan fasting in Saudi Arabia on serum bone profile and immunoglobulins', NCBI, October 2015, https://www.ncbi.nlm.nih.gov/pmc/articles/PMC4579416/

43. Papagiannopoulos I.A., Sideris V.I., Boschmann M., Koutsoni O.S. and Dotsika E.N., 'Anthropometric, Hemodynamic, Metabolic, and Renal Responses during 5 Days of Food and Water Deprivation', Karger, December 2013, https://www.karger.com/Article/Abstract/357718

44. Ca layan EK, Göçmen AY and Delibas N, 'Effects of long-term fasting on female hormone levels: Ramadan model', NCBI, https://www.ncbi.nlm.nih.gov/pubmed/24707675

45. Fereidoun Azizi, 'Islamic Fasting and Thyroid Hormones', NCBI, 25 April 2015, https://www.ncbi.nlm.nih.gov/pmc/articles/PMC4450165/

46. Syed A. Raza, Osama Ishtiaq, A.G. Unnikrishnan, A.K. Azad Khan, Jamal Ahmad, Mohammed A. Ganie, Kishwar Azad, Manash Baruah and Md Faruque Pathan, 'Thyroid diseases and Ramadan', NCBI, July–August 2012, https://www.ncbi.nlm.nih.gov/pmc/articles/PMC3401749/

47. The National Academy of Hypothyroidism, 'What Is Intermittent Fasting and Is It Safe for Thyroid Patients?', Nahis, 6 September 2018, https://www.nahypothyroidism.org/what-is-intermittent-fasting-and-is-it-safe-for-thyroid-patients/#

48. Kamel S. Kamel, Shih-Hua Lin, Surinder Cheema-Dhadli, Errol B. Marliss and Mitchell L. Halperin, 'Prolonged total fasting: A feast for the integrative physiologist', Kidney International, Vol. 53 (1998), pp. 531–539, https://www.kidney-international.org/article/S0085-2538(15)60426-4/pdf

49. Dr Randi Fredricks, PhD, 'Dry Fasting', Natural Mental Health Care, 12 July 2008, http:// naturalmentalhealthcare.net/dry-fasting/

50. Ruth E. Patterson, PhD, Gail A. Laughlin, PhD, Dorothy D. Sears, PhD, Andrea Z. LaCroix, PhD, Catherine Marinac, BA, Linda C. Gallo, PhD, Sheri J. Hartman, PhD, Loki Natarajan, PhD, Carolyn M. Senger, MD, María Elena Martínez, PhD and Adriana Villaseñor, PhD, 'Intermittent Fasting and Human Metabolic Health', NCBI, 6 April 2015, https://www. ncbi.nlm.nih.gov/pmc/articles/PMC4516560/

51. 'Fasting Quotes, Historical and Modern Day Quotes on the Value of Fasting', All About Fasting, https:// www.allaboutfasting.com/fasting-quotes.html

52. 'A little starvation can really do more for the average sick man than can the best medicines and the best doctors', Mark Twain, 'Autobiography of Mark Twain, Volume 1: The Complete and Authoritative Edition', University of California Press, 2010, p. 137, https://www.azquotes.com/quote/796775